Hypoactive Sexual Desire Disorder

Elena Vittoria Longhi

Hypoactive Sexual Desire Disorder

Psychosexological Overview for Clinicians

Springer

Elena Vittoria Longhi
Sexual Medical Center
San Raffaele Hospital
Milano, Italy

ISBN 978-3-032-00658-5 ISBN 978-3-032-00659-2 (eBook)
https://doi.org/10.1007/978-3-032-00659-2

The original submitted manuscript has been translated into English. The translation was done using artificial intelligence. A subsequent revision was performed by the author(s) to further refine the work and to ensure that the translation is appropriate concerning content and scientific correctness. It may, however, read stylistically different from a conventional translation.

This Springer imprint is published by the registered company Springer Nature Switzerland AG
The registered company address is: Gewerbestrasse 11, 6330 Cham, Switzerland

Foreword by Sara Baldini and Federico Dehò

Male Hypoactive Sexual Desire Disorder (HSDD) presents one of the most intricate challenges in andrological, endocrinological, and psychosexual clinical practice. Often overlooked or erroneously attributed solely to psychological factors, HSDD actually stems from a multifactorial interaction involving biological, neuroendocrine, relational, and sociocultural aspects. The imbalance between these factors can significantly impact both individual and couple' quality of life. The lack of a standardized diagnostic and therapeutic framework, coupled with often ineffective communication between physician and patient, further complicates the management of this condition.

This volume aims to equip healthcare professionals with a comprehensive and scientifically grounded perspective. In this regard, it offers a systematic and up-to-date review of the international scientific literature, integrating the guidelines of the DSM-5 and the International Society for the Study of Women's Sexual Health with the latest clinical evidence. Through a systemic and interdisciplinary approach, the book also delves into the less frequently studied variants of sexual desire disorders, such as hypersexuality, asexuality, and sexual aversion, highlighting their unique etiological and therapeutic aspects. This expanded perspective on HSDD allows for a deeper understanding of the disorder's psychopathological and somatic implications across different patient cohorts.

Particular attention is given to diagnostic tools, including the Sexual Desire Relationship Distress Scale (SDRDS) and the Sexual Interest and Desire Inventory-Female (SIDI-F), as well as therapeutic options ranging from pharmacological treatments to psychological and behavioral interventions. The book provides a clear overview of current treatment strategies, emphasizing the differences in clinical presentation and therapeutic approaches between men and women: while male HSDD is often addressed with targeted hormonal or pharmacological interventions, in women, the disorder is more strongly influenced by psychological and relational factors, necessitating a multidimensional management approach.

Beyond clinical aspects, the volume also explores relevant social and cultural issues, such as the role of body image, cross-cultural differences in physician-patient communication, and the impact of HSDD in specific populations, including patients with opioid dependence, veterans with post-traumatic stress disorder, and individuals with chronic conditions such as diabetes, multiple sclerosis, and polycystic ovary syndrome. The goal is to move beyond reductive interpretations and promote a therapeutic approach tailored to the patient's actual needs.

This book is intended for specialists, researchers, and healthcare professionals in the field of sexual medicine, providing practical clinical tools for the diagnostic and therapeutic management of HSDD. We hope that it will contribute to improving patient care and foster a more comprehensive understanding of male sexuality.

Urology Resident, ASST Sette Laghi – Sara Baldini
Circolo & Fondazione Macchi Hospital
Varese, Italy
University of Insubria
Varese, Italy

Director of Urology Department Federico Dehò
ASST Sette Laghi – Circolo & Fondazione Macchi Hospital
Varese, Italy
Associate Professor of Urology
Director of Urology Residency Program
University of Insubria
Varese, Italy

Foreword by Ida Bianchessi

The Pinkus contraceptive pill in 1968 and the advent of sildenafil in 1998 revolutionized sexual customs worldwide. Pharmacologically induced erections largely solved the problem of erectile dysfunction, and andrologists believed there were no longer any obstacles to a good sexual relationship. Meanwhile, in the globalized world, the term "performance" was increasingly used instead of "intimate relationship" or "making love." Female desire disorders, known for millennia and labeled as frigidity, were now highlighted by the blue pill, which brought male libido disorders into focus. But what do we mean by desire disorders, or HSDD? The DSM-5 includes them among pathologies only if the absence or decreased sexual desire causes distress. Therefore, if an individual does not feel sexual desire and has other interests that fully satisfy them in life, the absence of sexual desire is not considered pathological. The problem, in this case, reflects on the partner, if the individual is in a relationship, because it causes distress in the partner who would like a sexual relationship. But let's see what the lack of libido means for the patient: often the patient, unlike the andrologist, identifies desire with arousal, with stimulus, with the erection itself as they equate cause with effect—I desire therefore I have an erection, I have an erection therefore I desire, I have libido. Of course, for the specialist, who has conducted a thorough analysis of the physiological, biochemical, and psychological process of the phenomenon, it is not so. Simply put, desire is the always half-empty glass that one wants to fill. I have noticed another peculiarity of the disorder, it is not characteristic of the older patient who typically says "I would like to but I can't." HSDD in females is often secondary to years of frustration due to the partner's premature ejaculation, which triggers the cascade of arousal, concluding the sexual act before the woman can reach orgasm, causing a strong sense of pleasure denial, sometimes accompanied by pelvic pain. In males, it can appear after prostatitis, or active phase Induratio Penis Plastica, or trauma outcomes, always due to the presence of a painful component. HSDD, which has been accompanying us for 30 years in our clinics, increasingly begins as an indifference to sexuality, a vague discomfort at the idea of intimacy, couples attribute the cause to lack of time. What is not explained is why, if technology helps to make everything faster and easier, partners have less time to be together, they should have more; this is precisely the point: technological tools are no longer the means but become the end, the object that completely absorbs us, at work, in friendship, in affection, in every form of communication for better or worse. Young people get used to having everything immediately, they don't have time to desire, and it is the lack and the wait that feed, together with fantasy, the desire. The world of images that surrounds us leaves no space for imagination, the passivity to which the screen subjugates us, sterilizes our imagination, while in fragile minds it can lead to obsession, to addiction. The screen feeds us models of men and women who are unreachable, perfect, plastic, lips, breasts, buttocks, legs, arms, all the same. Individuality, the uniqueness of the individual, begins to be lacking. There is a sort of "globalization of bodies" where the woman enjoys pleasing and being pleased as an image but often fails to experience physical pleasure, the man is dazzled by the image and often develops performance anxiety. This volume seeks to respond to the contradictions of our time not only with an overview of the literature on desire disorders but with the field experience of a sexologist who for decades has integrated and supported the work of urologists and andrologists for hundreds of patients.

Medical Surgeon – Specialist in Urology – Ida Bianchessi
Clinical Andro-sexologist
Former Head of the Division of Urology –
I.R.C.C.S. Policlinico S. Matteo-Pavia
Pavia, Italy

Former Consultant Spinal Unit Fondazione Maugeri Pavia
Pavia, Italy

Foreword by Carlo Ceruti

There are individuals who have the gift of facilitating dialogue between different worlds, professionals who can intuit which skills are unique to a particular sector that could be useful to transfer to professionals from different cultural backgrounds and at the same time capable of promoting this transfer of knowledge through the use of a common language.

I have always considered Elena Longhi a prominent representative of this category: as a urologist and andrologist, hearing her talk about sexology is a continuous discovery not of a distant and separate world, but of an adjacent aspect, often complementary to our professional field, yet rarely brought to light. A very practical sexology, that helps to better understand patients, that explains the reasons behind things.

This book will also make us reflect and will help us in knowing how to be, more and more, the doctor that our patients would like to find.

Carlo Ceruti

Senior Consultant Urologist and Andrologist
Assistant Professor in Urology and Coordinator
of Master in Andrology
Turin, Italy

City of Health and Science Hospital
University of Turin
Turin, Italy

Preface

Hypoactive sexual desire disorder (HSDD) is a dysfunction that affects and disturbs individuals, couples, and even clinicians.

The complexity of this disorder is not age related: even young people, often dependent on the use of mass media and pornography, report a physical, psychological state of sexual inactivity, due to lack of desire or total or partial absence of sexual fantasies.

This condition encompasses multiple factors: biological, psychological, gender-related, relational, and social in general.

Andrologists and gynecologists investigate the biological causes through blood tests, hormonal tests, etc., but often a neuropsychological or psychosexual component is hypothesized only in the absence of exemplary clinical data.

In my clinical career, I have encountered individuals and couples troubled by the fact that they were free from underlying clinical pathologies. The idea among patients that the psychological cause does not refer to a psychiatric pathology but to the complexity of the person, not investigable with blood markers, is still not widespread.

In the Sexual Medicine Center, where I have been working since 2000, in collaboration with andrologists, urologists, and specialists from every hospital department, we have tried to set up a team approach where diagnosis and treatment depend on the clinical picture and sexual anamnesis.

The chapters of this text aim to provide a broader picture of hypoactive desire disorder, involving clinical studies on the subject, our field research, and information suggested by patients.

The text does not intend to be a manual, rather a journey through the various aspects of a disorder that affects the quality of life of the patient and the couple.

An encouragement to look beyond basic orthodoxy and to deepen the curiosity of clinicians and students toward a systemic view beyond the manual.

Specialist in Family Therapy, Sexology
Psycho-oncology, Center for Sexual Medicine
U.O Urology-Vita & Salute University
Milan, Italy

Elena Vittoria Longhi

Introduction

The Labyrinth of Sexual Desire

The World Association of Sexual Health (WAS) has recently defined sexual pleasure as "the physical and/or psychological satisfaction and enjoyment derived from shared or solitary erotic experiences, including thoughts, fantasies, dreams, emotions, and feelings" [1]. But what about desire?

According to the incentive motivation model, sexual desire is activated by external stimuli that are sexually relevant or by mental representations of such stimuli [2]. This conceptualization of sexual desire contrasts with that of many other researchers who, influenced by Freud [3] and Kaplan [4], consider sexual desire to originate internally, as a drive that awakens "spontaneously" through deprivation.

Consequently, the vast majority of questionnaires used in clinical practice and research to quantify sexual desire are based on the assumption that sexual desire is a stable trait, a capacity that one either possesses or does not, and is often claimed to be stronger in men than in women.

It is interesting to note that studies using self-report questionnaires that conceptualize sexual desire consistently find gender differences in the stereotypical direction (with men reporting higher desire), while studies in which individuals assess their feelings of sexual desire immediately after exposure to a sexual stimulus fail to find differences between women and men [5]. However, even recent studies using measures of sexual desire traits have questioned the idea that men have a high and unwavering sexual desire [6].

The almost universal idea that men have higher levels of desire than women, that it is an innate capacity, is an idea reinforced by evolutionary theories and reproductive strategies, which may depend on how sexual desire is conceptualized and measured. If sexual desire is seen as emerging rather than preceding "incentivized" sexual arousal, gender differences in reported desire feelings may be the result of differences in the quality of the incentive or sexual context rather than a reflection of individual differences.

Sexual Desire and Hormones

The fact that men have 10–20 times more testosterone, expressed in absolute levels, compared to women [7], has often been mistakenly equated with the idea that men have a stronger innate sexual desire that increases in response to deprivation [8].

However, there is no evidence of increased sexual desire from sexual abstinence, and abstinence does not lead to life-threatening effects compared, for example, to a hunger or thirst strike [9]. If anything, in both women and men, the absence of partnered and/or solo sexual activity, or the presence of ungratifying sexual activity, seems to correlate with a reduction in the desire to be sexually active, with sexual abstinence even leading to reduced testosterone levels after prolonged periods of abstinence [10]. Even though a certain level of testosterone is necessary for men's brains and genitals to be sensitive to sexual stimuli, normal physiological levels of testosterone above that minimum threshold seem not to be correlated with levels of sexual desire [11].

The same might be true for women, for whom testosterone is also thought to be associated with their sexual excitability [12]. As in men, it is possible that in women testosterone is not linearly but curvilinearly related to sexual function across the entire serum T range. This implies that androgen-related sexual problems should only be anticipated when T levels are below a certain hypo-physiological threshold, yet to be determined.

Supporting a threshold approach, a recent study on women infected with the human immunodeficiency virus showed that self-reported problems with sexual desire and other androgen-related symptoms such as depression, fatigue, and reduced physical functionality were higher in women with T deficiency compared to those without (with T deficiency defined as total $T \leq 0.3$ if sex hormone-binding globulin (SHBG) levels were in the normal range (<100 nmol/L) and as total $T \times [100 * T/\text{SHBG}] \leq 0.5$ in patients with elevated SHBG levels) [13]. In short, it is not absolute hormonal levels but rather relative ones that may enable women and men to be sensitive to sexual stimulation.

Is Desire a Matter of the Mind?

Key brain regions that regulate sexual desire include the prefrontal cortex, the locus coeruleus, the medial preoptic area, the paraventricular nucleus, and the reward and attention processing centers of the ventral tegmental area and the nucleus accumbens [14]. Sexual arousal involves the actions of brain dopamine, melanocortin, oxytocin, vasopressin, and noradrenaline [15]. These neurotransmitters coordinate pathways in the hypothalamus, limbic system, and cortex to process and respond to sexual stimuli. Sexual inhibition involves the opioid, serotonin, and endocannabinoid systems, brain areas that are normally activated during sexual refractoriness or in response to primary aversion or secondary avoidance.

A broad scientific literature on the psychopharmacology of sexual motivation and desire reports that sexual desire can be inhibited by drugs or conditions that:

1. Decrease dopamine levels in the brain
2. Increase the action of serotonin in the brain specifically through serotonin 2A receptors
3. Increase opioids that act on mu receptors

Conversely, sexual desire can be stimulated by drugs or conditions that:

1. Increase hypothalamic and mesolimbic dopamine
2. Decrease the release of serotonin or inhibit postsynaptic binding in the prefrontal cortex

Drugs that can selectively activate these stimulatory pathways or reduce inhibitory pathways are actively being evaluated for the treatment of hypoactive sexual desire disorder (HSDD), with one (flibanserin) currently approved by the Food and Drug Administration (FDA) [16].

Milan, Italy Elena Vittoria Longhi

References

1. World Association of Sexual Health. Declaration on sexual pleasure. 2019. https://worldsexualhealth.net/declaration-on-sexual-pleasure.
2. Toates F. How sexual desire works: the enigmatic urge. Cambridge University Press; 2014.
3. Freud S. Three essays on the theory of sexuality. In: Strachey J, editor. The standard edition of the complete psychological works of Sigmund Freud. Hogarth Press; 1953 (Original work published in 1905).
4. Kaplan HS. The sexual desire disorders. Dysfunctional regulation of sexual motivation. Brunner and Mazel; 1995.
5. Dawson SJ, Chivers ML. Gender-specificity of solitary and dyadic sexual desire among gynephilic and androphilic women and men. J Sexual Med. 2014; 11(4): 980–94.
6. Murray SH. Not always in the mood: the new science of men, sex, and relationships. Rowman & Littlefield; 2019.
7. Wang Y, Gay GD, Botelho JC, Caudill SP, Vesper HW. Total testosterone quantitative measurement in serum by LC-MS/MS. Clinica Chimica Acta. 2014; 436: 263–7. https://doi.org/10.1016/j.cca.2014.06.009.
8. Kaplan HS. The sexual desire disorders. Dysfunctional regulation of sexual motivation. Brunner and Mazel; 1995.
9. Both S, Everaerd W, Laan E. Desire emerges from excitement: a psychophysiological perspective on sexual motivation. In Janssen E, editor. The psychophysiology of sex. Indiana University Press; 2007. pp. 327–39.
10. Hsu B, Cumming RG, Blyth FM, Naganathan V, Le Couteur DG, Seibel MJ, Waite LM, Handelsman DJ. The longitudinal relationship of sexual function and androgen status in older men: the Concord Health and Ageing in Men Project. J Clin Endocrinol Metabol. 2015; 4: 1350–8.

11. Rastrelli G, Corona G, Maggi M. Testosterone and sexual function in men. Maturitas. 2018; 112: 46–52. https://doi.org/10.1016/j.maturitas.2018.04.004.
12. Le Moëne O, Ågmo A. (2018). The neuroendocrinology of sexual attraction. Front Neuroendocrinol. 2018; 51: 46–67. https://doi.org/10.1016/j.yfrne.2017.12.006.
13. Laan E, van Lunsen HW, Prins JM, Nieuwkerk PT, Nievaard MAF. (2019). Testosterone insufficiency in human immunodeficiency virus-infected women: a cross-sectional study. Sexual Med. 2019; 7(1): 72–9. https://doi.org/10.1016/j.esxm.2018.10.002.
14. Pfaus JG. Pathways of sexual desire. J Sex Med. 2009; 6(6): 1506–33.
15. Steel SM. Targeting the circuits of sexual desire as a treatment strategy for hypoactive sexual desire disorder. J Clin Psychiatry. 2010, 71(7): 821–2.
16. Sale A, Berardi N, Maffei L. Environment and brain plasticity: towards an endogenous pharmacotherapy. Physiol Rev. 2014; 94(1): 189–234.

Contents

Part I

Foundations and Diagnostic Frameworks

Hypoactive Sexual Desire Disorder (HSDD): Guidelines for the Diagnostic and Statistical Manual of Mental Disorders (DSM-5) in Men and Women

1

Abstract

Many uncertainties about the differences between men and women in many aspects of sexual life remain to be understood. One of these is *compulsive sexual behavior disorder*, which continues to be more frequent in men, although neuroticism and vulnerability to stress are to be reported more frequently in women. But not least, *hypoactive sexual desire disorder*—in men and women. Further scientific research is increasingly necessary to deeply understand not only the differences but also the best approaches to overcome these disorders when they constitute barriers to understanding and enjoying the sexual experience.

Keywords

Diagnostic guidelines · Psychological causes · Relational · Chronic underlying pathologies · Couple conflicts · Ongoing scientific research · DSM

1.1 Introduction

Male and female hypoactive sexual desire disorder (HSDD), or low sexual desire with associated personal distress, is a clinical condition that has a negative impact on well-being, on quality of life, and on relationships. Low desire can involve a lack of motivation, desire, or interest in sexual activity, including the loss of responsive desire. Low desire is considered problematic or a dysfunction only if it is associated with substantial personal distress.

Although there is some overlap between HSDD and female sexual arousal disorder, for example, these entities differ in their etiologies, risk factors, clinical characteristics, and responses to psychological and pharmaceutical interventions. Documenting the prevalence of HSDD for epidemiological purposes is difficult since a clinical diagnosis requires a face-to-face evaluation to exclude factors that may be the primary cause of low desire.

E. V. Longhi, *Hypoactive Sexual Desire Disorder*,
https://doi.org/10.1007/978-3-032-00659-2_1

1.2 Theoretical References

In the Diagnostic and Statistical Manual of Mental Disorders (DSM) V-TR, hypoactive sexual desire disorder (HSDD) is defined as "*The persistent or recurrent lack or absence of sexual fantasies and desire for sexual activity with marked distress or interpersonal difficulty not otherwise explained by a general medical or psychiatric condition.*" ***HSDD can be primary or secondary, lifelong or acquired, and generalized or situational*** [1].

In DSM-5, HSDD and female sexual arousal disorder were combined into a single diagnosis: female sexual interest and arousal disorder [2].

Although HSDD may overlap with other sexual health disorders, it is a distinct diagnostic category. Based on this evidence, HSDD is the desire dysfunction specified in the ISSWSH nomenclature, in the classification of the Fourth International Consultation on Sexual Medicine, in the International Classification of Diseases, tenth edition (ICD-10), and in the upcoming International Classification of Diseases, 11th edition (ICD-11) [3].

It is believed that 1 in 10 women (and 1 in 15 men) may suffer from chronic hypoactive sexual desire disorder. The causes of low desire include chronic medical conditions, medications, surgical interventions, and psychosocial factors, but not advancing age; both pre- and postmenopausal women can have HSDD, as can young adult men or those over 50.

Sexual function requires the complex interaction of multiple neurotransmitters and hormones, both at the central and peripheral levels, and *sexual desire are considered the result of a complex balance between inhibitory and excitatory pathways in the brain*. For example, dopamine, estrogens, progesterone, and testosterone play an excitatory role, while serotonin and prolactin are inhibitors.

Therefore, a hypoactive sexual desire could be due to a reduced level of excitatory activity, an increased level of inhibitory activity, or both. In addition to individual psychological causes, relational and social factors also contribute. Several validated self-assessment and specialist-administered tools are available to assess the extent of desire. The ***Decreased Sexual Desire Screener*** (DSDS) was developed for specialists who are neither trained nor specialized in FSD to help make an accurate diagnosis of generalized and/or chronic acquired HSDD [4].

As early as the late 1990s, Basson [5] observed in patients seeking treatment and their sexually healthy partners that typically one or both partners initiated sexual intercourse for a variety of reasons, some of which were not related to the experience of sexual desire. This observation led Basson to propose a sexual response model in which *sexual desire was largely reactive in nature—that is, consequent to arousal, so much so that desire and arousal can be experienced simultaneously*.

The need for sexual stimuli in an appropriate, intimate context for each partner, the ability to stay focused on the moment (mood and other biological and psychological factors that influence the processing of sexual information), have been described in Basson's "*circular model.*"

In this reading, desire would not be the premise of a passionate, intimate experience, but the consequence of a momentary arousal of the couple in an enticing context.

1.3 A Creative Clinical Experience

The study by O'Loughlin et al. [6] recruited 324 participants in response to an advertisement targeted at women with low sexual desire: "*Are you a woman aged between 19 and 65 who has low or absent sexual desire?*" Women who responded to the advertisement and who met the inclusion criteria—age between 19 and 65 years, without known serious medical diseases that affect sexual functioning, who were not smokers, currently not depressed, and who did not use drugs with known side effects on sexual functioning (for example, antidepressants), nor topical or oral products based on dehydroepiandrosterone (DHEA), nor hormonal contraceptives, nor hormone replacement therapy—were provided with more information about the study.

The inclusion criteria were established to ensure consistency with the diagnosis of HSDD *from the DSM*-IV, and with the aim of eliminating factors known to disrupt the hormones measured in the larger study (for example, cortisol, DHEA). The ads were published online (for example, Craigslist, list of paid university students, hospital electronic mailing lists), in local newspapers, and on flyers posted throughout the community (for example, bus stops, university bulletin boards, hospital bulletin boards). Even family doctors who met patients with sexual problems were encouraged to post an ad in their own clinics.

The operational criteria for HSDD were evaluated through a telephone screening interview conducted by a qualified research assistant.

If the potential participant reported regular drug use, a body mass index (BMI) below 18.5 or above 29.9, an ongoing pregnancy, or stress levels that interfered with daily functions, *the telephone interview was terminated, and the respondent was thanked for their time*. In addition, women who reported low desire were excluded from participation if they experienced pain during intercourse, if the low sexual desire was directly associated with discord in the relationship, or if the low desire had been present for less than a year.

Respondents who met the inclusion criteria were emailed a consent form for the full study and asked for a face-to-face meeting with a research assistant to review the study procedures in more detail. After this meeting, each participant received via email a series of online questionnaires to self-complete; a hormonal sample was taken for the larger study, and a second face-to-face meeting with a clinical interviewer was scheduled to assess the HSDD criteria and confirm a diagnosis.

Participants received a monetary compensation of $100 for completing the questionnaires, interviews, and home hormonal collection. Partial compensation (from $25 to $75) was provided for incomplete participation.

1.4 Self-Completed Questionnaires

The self-completed questionnaires were: the *Decreased Sexual Desire Screener* (DSDS) [7], a short diagnostic screening tool of five questions; the *Reliability and validity of the Sexual Interest and Desire Inventory—Female* (SIDI-F) [8], a 13-item measure of sexual interest, desire, and excitability; and the SIAD [9].

1.4.1 Results

Of the 291 women who participated in this study, 151 met the criteria for HSDD, and 140 did not. Among the 151 women who met the criteria for HSDD, 111 also met the criteria for *Sexual Interest/Arousal Disorder* (SIAD) (73.5%), and 40 women did not (26.5%). Among the 140 women who did not meet the criteria for HSDD, none met the criteria for SIAD. This group served as a nonclinical control group.

Approximately 42.27% of the sample reported reduced interest in sexual activity; 32.50% reported a lack of sexual desire; 35.05% showed reduced or no erotic fantasies; 42.24% reported poor or no receptivity to the sexual invitations of their partner; 74.07% rated their sexual desire as little responsive to sexual stimuli; and 59.80% reported difficulties related to genital and/or non-genital sensations during sexual activity [10].

In the comparison between men and women, the study by Giraldi A et al. [11] recruited 499 men and 573 women. Only the responses of sexually active participants with a partner (401 men and 429 women) were analyzed. The *Female Sexual Function Index*, the *Female Sexual Distress Scale*, and the *International Index of Erectile Function* were used to describe sexual function. Additionally, participants completed questionnaires with written descriptions of various sexual responses to describe their most experienced sexual response. Among men, erectile dysfunction and dissatisfaction with sexual life were significantly correlated. Among women, lack of desire was linked to apathy toward erotic fantasies or external sexual stimuli. The lack of uniform diagnostic criteria—McCabe MP's study [12] recruited 741 women from Australia, the Americas, Europe, and Asia. The participants were aged between 18 and 71 years and were involved in a heterosexual relationship lasting between 3 months and 49 years. Sexual desire problems were defined using a variety of criteria, including: (1) meeting the DSM-IV-TR criteria for hypoactive sexual desire disorder (HSDD), (2) meeting the DSM-IV-TR criteria for HSDD, removing the requirement for sexual thoughts/fantasies, (3) self-identified "lack of sexual interest," and (4) low average ratings of sexual desire levels, as assessed using the *Female Sexual Desire Questionnaire*. The prevalence of sexual desire problems varied from 3.0% to 31.0% depending on the criteria used to define such problems. It is important to reach a consensus on the criteria used to define sexual desire problems in order to standardize and compare studies investigating these issues. The way women's sexual desire problems are conceptualized has implications for their treatment. Therapists may or may not need to address absent sexual thoughts/

fantasies and may work with low normative levels of desire versus subjective ratings of low desire. Lack of interest in sex is a common sexual problem among women and men, and it may be associated with less relational satisfaction and greater psychological distress. Research on sexual motivation has shown that, in both clinical and community samples, people with a higher communal sexual strength (motivated to meet the sexual needs of their partner) and approach sexual goals (motivated to engage in sex to pursue positive outcomes) report greater desire and relational satisfaction, while people with avoidance sexual goals (motivated to engage in sex to avoid negative outcomes) tend to report lower desire and satisfaction. In the study by Bockaj A. [13], the sexual motivation of women diagnosed with *female sexual interest/arousal disorder* (*FSIAD*), who reported chronically low desire and arousal accompanied by discomfort, and their partners ($N = 97$ couples) was compared with couples without sexual dysfunction ($N = 108$ couples). Women with FSIAD reported lower communal sexual strength and approach goals and higher avoidance sexual goals compared to control women and their partners. However, the partners of women with FSIAD did not report differences in sexual motivation compared to control partners. Sexual motivation could be a target for future intervention studies on couples facing problems of low desire and poor arousal.

1.4.2 Conclusions

It was found that women with HSDD have a compromised body image, self-esteem, and self-worth, and feel less connected to their partners [14]. Total healthcare costs, compared to a control patient cohort, were higher for women with HSDD, including outpatient visits, prescription drug use, and other medical services such as radiology, laboratory work, and outpatient procedures [15]. Comorbidities include depression and fatigue, similar to chronic conditions such as diabetes and back pain [16]. Research on the central neuroendocrine mechanisms of sexual desire has led to a better understanding of the underlying pathogenesis of this biopsychosocial condition. Despite numerous publications on HSDD, what has been lacking is a concise resource to assist clinicians (internists, general practitioners, gynecologists, urologists, and advanced practice providers) in competently screening patients for HSDD and providing appropriate therapeutic options within a biopsychosocial paradigm. To this end, the *International Society for the Study of Women's Sexual Health* (ISSWSH) commissioned a group of experts to draft a concise review of the neural circuit that regulates sexual desire, including a plausible explanation for persistent states of both normal and hypoactive sexual desire; a description of current on-label and off-label treatment strategies, including their benefits and pitfalls; and a discussion on the rationale for using various therapies.

In January 2016, the executive committee of the ISSWSH (a multidisciplinary academic and scientific non-profit organization dedicated to supporting the highest standards of ethics and professionalism in research, education, and clinical practice of sexual health) chose the co-chairs for this project to identify potential speakers based on individual publications and research. The group of 13 researchers and clinicians met in Dallas, Texas, to present and discuss the current state of knowledge on HSDD.

It was defined that the treatment of HSDD may involve both psychosocial and biological strategies, since psychosocial/interpersonal and biological factors influence each other [17]. However, it is reasonable to prepare an individualized treatment plan, taking into account the most distressing factors for that particular patient. A brief outpatient consultation can be useful, using the PLISSIT model (Permission, Limited Information, Specific Suggestions, and Intensive Therapy), in addition to the indication of a more appropriate sexological therapy.

The study by Ertl N et al. [18] delved into the "*top-down*" *theory of HSDD*, which describes hyperactivity in higher-level cognitive brain regions, suppressing lower-level emotional and sexual brain areas. However, it is not known how this neurofunctional disorder compares with HSDD in men versus women. To investigate this hypothesis, researchers used functional magnetic resonance imaging based on activity in 32 women and 32 men with HSDD to measure the brain's sexual processing during sexual videos compared to non-sexual ones, as well as psychometric questionnaires to assess sexual desire and arousal. It was shown that women had greater activation in both higher- and lower-level brain regions compared to men. In fact, *women who exhibited greater hypothalamic activation in response to sexual videos reported higher psychometric scores in the evaluative, motivational, and physiological domains of sexual desire and arousal after watching the sexual videos in the scanner*. However, no similar correlations were observed in men. Overall, this is the first direct comparison of the neural correlates of low and distressing sexual desire between women and men. ***The data support the "top-down" theory of HSDD in women, while in men; HSDD seems to be associated with different neurofunctional processes.***

On the other hand, the study by Stoléru S et al. [19] identified, in patients with *hypoactive sexual desire disorder* (HSDD), the brain regions where functional disturbances disrupt the regulation of sexual motivation. Positron emission tomography was used to compare seven male patients with HSDD with eight healthy men on their regional responses of cerebral blood flow to graded-intensity visual sexual stimuli (VSS).

Statistical parametric mapping was used to identify the brain regions that showed differential activation (or deactivation) in the groups. While in control subjects the medial orbitofrontal cortex showed deactivation in response to VSS, *in patients with HSDD, there was abnormally maintained activity in this region, which has been implicated in the inhibitory control of motivated behavior.* Conversely, the inverse model (activation in control subjects, deactivation or unchanged activity in patients) was found in the secondary somatosensory cortex and the inferior parietal lobules—regions that mediate the processes of emotional and motor imagination—as well as in those areas of the anterior cingulate gyrus and the frontal lobes involved in premotor processes.

References

1. McCabe M, Sharlip ID, Atalla E, et al. Definitions of sexual dysfunctions in women and men: a consensus statement from the fourth international consultation on sexual medicine. J Sex Med. 2015;13:135–43.
2. American Psychological Association. Diagnostic and statistical manual of mental disorders (fifth edition: DSM-5). Arlington: American Psychological Association; 2013.
3. Reed GM, Drescher J, Krueger RB, et al. Disorders related to sexuality and gender identity in the ICD-11: revision of the ICD-10 classification based on current scientific evidence, best clinical practices, and human rights considerations. World Psychiatry. 2016;15:205–21.
4. Simon JA. Low sexual desire: is it all in your head? Pathophysiology, diagnosis, and treatment of hypoactive sexual desire disorder. Postgrad Med. 2010;122(6):128–36. https://doi.org/10.3810/pgm.2010.11.2230.
5. Basson R. Human sex-response cycles. J Sex Marital Ther. 2001;27:33–43. https://doi.org/10.1080/00926230152035831.
6. O'Loughlin JI, Basson R, Brotto LA. Women with hypoactive sexual desire disorder versus sexual interest/arousal disorder: an empirical test for raising the bar. J Sex Res. 2017;55(6):734–46. https://doi.org/10.1080/00224499.2017.1386764.
7. Clayton AH, Goldfischer ER, Goldstein I, DeRogatis L, Lewis-D'Agostino DJ, Pyke R. Validation of the decreased sexual desire screener (DSDS): a brief diagnostic instrument for generalized acquired female hypoactive sexual desire disorder (HSDD). J Sex Med. 2009;6:730–8. https://doi.org/10.1111/j.1743-6109.2008.01153.x.
8. Clayton AH, Segraves RT, Leiblum S, Basson R, Pyke R, Cotton D, et al. Reliability and validity of the sexual interest and desire inventory—female (SIDI-F), a scale designed to measure severity of female hypoactive sexual desire disorder. J Sex Marital Ther. 2006;32:115–35. https://doi.org/10.1080/00926230500442300.
9. American Psychiatric Association. Diagnostic and statistical manual of mental disorders. 5th ed. Arlington: American Psychiatric Publishing; 2013.
10. Carvalheira AA, Brotto LA, Leal I. Women's motivations for sex: exploration of the diagnostic and statistical manual, text revision criteria for hypoactive sexual desire and female sexual arousal disorders. J Sex Med. 2010;7:1454–63. https://doi.org/10.1111/j.1743-6109.2009.01693.x.
11. Giraldi A, Kristensen E, Sand M. Endorsement of models describing sexual response of men and women with a sexual partner: an online survey in a population sample of Danish adults ages 20–65 years. J Sex Med. 2015;12(1):116–28. https://doi.org/10.1111/jsm.12720. Epub 2014 Nov 3. PMID: 25363341
12. McCabe MP, Goldhammer DL. Prevalence of women's sexual desire problems: what criteria do we use? Arch Sex Behav. 2013;42(6):1073–8. https://doi.org/10.1007/s10508-013-0107-z. Epub 2013 May 15. PMID: 23674067.
13. Bockaj A, Rosen NO, Muise A. Sexual motivation in couples facing female sexual interest/arousal disorder: a comparison with control couples. J Sex Marital Ther. 2019;45(8):796–808. https://doi.org/10.1080/0092623X.2019.1623356.
14. Kingsberg, South Africa. Survey on the attitudes of women living with low sexual desire. J Women's Health (Larchmt). 2014;23(10):817–23.
15. Foley F. Healthcare resource use and expenditures of women diagnosed with hypoactive sexual desire disorder. J Med Econ. 2010;13(4):583–90.
16. Biddle AK, West SL, D'Aloisio AA, Wheeler SB, Borisov NN, Thorp J. Hypoactive sexual desire disorder in postmenopausal women: quality of life and impact on health. Health Value. 2009;12(5):763–72.
17. Brotto L, Atallah S, Johnson-Agbakwu C, et al. Psychological and interpersonal dimensions of sexual function and dysfunction. J Sex Med. 2016;13(4):538–71.

18. Ertl N, Mills EG, Wall MB, Thurston L, Yang L, Suladze S, Hunjan T, Phylactou M, Patel B, Bassett PA, Howard J, Rabiner EA, Abbara A, Goldmeier D, Comninos AN, Dhillo WS. Women and men with distressing low sexual desire exhibit sexually dimorphic brain processing. Sci Rep. 2024;14(1):11051. https://doi.org/10.1038/s41598-024-61190-4. PMID: 38745001; PMCID: PMC11094107.
19. Stoléru S, Redouté J, Costes N, Lavenne F, Bars DL, Dechaud H, Forest MG, Pugeat M, Cinotti L, Pujol JF. Brain processing of visual sexual stimuli in men with hypoactive sexual desire disorder. Psychiatry Res. 2003;124(2):67–86. PMID: 14561426.

Hypoactive Sexual Desire Disorder and the Guidelines of the International Society for the Study of Sexual Health in Young and Adult Patients

2

Abstract

Sexual desire is one of the most common dysfunctions related to sexual health, especially in women, although differences in men have not been extensively studied. Among women, interpersonal problems and poor physical attraction are highly correlated with sexual interest: physical attraction and couple relational issues appear to be significant conditions of low sexual desire in women. Females, more often than males, seek psychosexual and psychological interventions, and both consider gynecologists and andrologists as the preferred professionals to consult.

Keywords

Hypoactive sexual desire in women and men · Medical therapies · Sexological therapies · Causes of HSDD

2.1 Introduction

The care process (POC) of the International Society for the Study of Women's Sexual Health for the management of *hypoactive sexual desiredisorder* (HSDD) was developed to provide evidence-based guidelines for the diagnosis and treatment of HSDD in women by healthcare professionals. Affecting **10% of adult women**, HSDD is associated with negative emotional and psychological states as well as medical conditions, including depression. Seventeen international speakers were recruited, representing multiple clinical disciplines. The POC begins with the healthcare professional asking for information about sexual concerns, focusing on issues related to low sexual desire of interest. The diagnosis includes distinguishing between generalized acquired HSDD and other forms of low sexual interest. The biopsychosocial assessment of potentially modifiable factors facilitates the start of treatment with education, modification of potentially modifiable factors, and, if

E. V. Longhi, *Hypoactive Sexual Desire Disorder*,
https://doi.org/10.1007/978-3-032-00659-2_2

necessary, further therapeutic intervention—such as sexual therapy, central nervous system agents, and hormonal therapy—partly guided by menopausal status. Sexual therapy includes behavioral therapy, cognitive-behavioral therapy, and mindfulness.

The only central nervous system agent currently approved by the U.S. Food and Drug Administration (FDA) for HSDD is flibanserin in premenopausal women; the use of flibanserin in postmenopausal women with HSDD is supported by data but is not FDA approved. Hormonal therapy includes the off-label use of testosterone in postmenopausal women with HSDD, supported by data but not FDA approved. The POC incorporates monitoring of therapy progress.

In summary, the POC of the International Society for the Study of Women's Sexual Health for the management of women with HSDD provides a rational, evidence-based guideline for healthcare professionals to manage patients with appropriate assessments and individualized treatments [1].

2.2 Scientific Research

Considering recent research and growing scientific awareness of HSDD, it is hypothesized that an increasing number of women will seek treatment for HSDD from a healthcare professional (HCP). This POC model consists of an evidence-based approach for identification, diagnosis, and treatment, which emphasizes bio-psychosocial assessment and education. It highlights opportunities to address modifiable factors, includes patient needs and preferences in the decision-making process, and defines situations for specialized referral.

The model incorporates the following essential principles:

1. Identification of HSDD subtypes (e.g., generalized versus situational and acquired versus lifelong), with emphasis on associated concurrent medical and psychological factors.
2. Importance of patient and partner coaching throughout all stages of management.
3. Goal-oriented approach with patient and partner needs and preferences guiding treatment recommendations.
4. Clear guidelines for follow-up and consideration of referral.

Clinical experience teaches that women with persistent and recurring disinterest in sexual activity report the absence of sexual fantasies and discomfort regarding a low, distressing sexual desire [2].

Furthermore, the ISSWSH [3] states that HSDD manifests for a minimum of 6 months with:

- Lack of motivation for sexual activity.
- Decreased or absent spontaneous desire (sexual thoughts or fantasies).
- Decrease or absence of responsive desire to erotic stimuli and signals or inability to maintain desire or interest through sexual activity.

- Loss of desire to initiate or participate in sexual activity, including behavioral responses such as avoidance of situations that could lead to sexual activity, which are not secondary to sexual pain disorders.
- Presence of frustration, distress, guilt, incompetence, loss, sadness, regret, or worry.

2.3 Research Questionnaires

Among the diagnostic tools, the **DSDS** is a validated questionnaire to confirm the diagnosis of *HSDD*: it is short, effective, easy to use, self-administered, and does not require any special training for administration and interpretation [4]. It includes five simple yes/no questions.

The first four questions incorporate the prerequisites for a diagnosis of generalized acquired HSDD: (A) previous satisfaction with their sexual desire/interest, (B) a decrease compared to previous satisfaction, (C) discomfort due to decreased sexual desire, and (D) desire to improve their sexual desire [5].

The majority of "no" answers would seem consistent with low sexual desire/interest throughout life. In the fifth question, the patient is asked to identify with yes/no answers which, if present, of the seven groups of factors listed could apply to their situation, potentially having a negative effect on their sexual desire/interest [6]. For example: (a surgical procedure, an unsatisfactory couple relationship, depression …).

If a patient answers "no" to at least one of the first four questions, they do not meet the criteria for generalized acquired HSDD but could meet the criteria for situational or permanent low sexual desire/interest.

If the patient answers "yes" to questions 1–4 and "no" to all the factors in question 5, they have generalized acquired HSDD.

If any of the factors in question 5 are present, clinicians can evaluate and consider differential diagnoses, including biological etiologies of low desire, as well as decide whether the answers to question 5 indicate generalized acquired HSDD or situational low sexual desire/interest. *Situational loss of desire can occur in response to a temporary stressful life situation*. Individuals with little or no sexual interest throughout their life, and who are not distressed, may be **asexual** and, as such, do not meet the criteria for HSDD, and no intervention is indicated [7], except for a psychosexual consultation.

As always, the sexual anamnesis should investigate the quality of emotional and sexual relationships over time (from adolescence to the present), family history (abortions, hereditary diseases, losses, abuses, abortions, …), the relationship with one's own body, the relationship developed with the opposite sex (separations, relationships with married partners, children, infertility, …), the acquired sexual education, and the predominant gender (heterosexual, bisexual, homosexual, queer, …).

Another diagnostic tool could be **the HCP**: it investigates poor motivation to participate in sexual activity, loss of spontaneous sexual desire (including sexual thoughts and fantasies), lack of desire in response to erotic stimuli and signals, poor initiative and avoidance of situations that could lead to sexual activity, and participation in sexual activity out of obligation or fear of losing the partner. It can include past and present characteristics of the patient's sexual desire/interest and other aspects of sexual function, such as arousal, orgasmic function, and/or any pain or discomfort during sexual activity.

2.4 The Causes of HSDD

Sexual function can be evaluated in relation to sexual activity with or without a partner and can include the history of sexual relationships with past and present partners. If there is a discrepancy in sexual desire between the patient and their partner, it can be considered HSDD only if the discrepancy in desire causes them discomfort. It should not be overlooked that sexual dysfunction could affect the patient's self-esteem and adaptability, as well as their social and professional performance [3].

The evaluation for HSDD should also include screening to assess arousal, orgasm, and the existence of pelvic pain to define a possible relationship between the onset of these disorders and low desire. It is also necessary to determine whether HSDD is permanent, acquired, and generalized or situational. In addition, investigating previous sexual functioning and relational/interpersonal problems is important [44–47]. It is important to note that a woman may experience HSDD and not have a stable relationship or have casual sexual partners[19].

The study called ***hypoactive sexual desire disorder registry for women***, with American patients with generalized acquired HSDD, highlighted arousal disorders, lubrication problems (or both), in 50.2%, 42.5%, and 39% of women with HSDD [8, 9].

Sleep problems, particularly insomnia, are common concerns among women. In the observational *Women's Health Initiative* study, higher insomnia scores and shorter sleep durations (<7 or 8 h) were associated with a reduction in sexual function. Improving the duration and quality of sleep can positively affect sexual function.

Also, **depression** affects sexual dysfunction, and antidepressant medications can be a cause or a potential adverse effect that may lead to discontinuation of treatment and a compromise in quality of life [10].

It is unlikely that targeted sexual therapy for HSDD will be effective if relational issues contributing to low desire or as a result of HSDD (for example, power, control, trust) are not addressed in patients with a dysfunctional partner or women with a history of sexual, physical, or emotional abuse.

2.5 Drugs that Act on the CNS and Hormonal Therapies

Among pharmacological treatments, **flibanserin** is currently the only drug approved by the U.S. Food and Drug Administration for acquired generalized HSDD in premenopausal women. This molecule (100 mg administered before retiring) is a daily, oral, multifunctional, centrally acting, nonhormonal serotonin agonist and antagonist. Three studies with a sample of more than 3500 patients showed a significant improvement in sexual desire and in the number of sexually satisfying events [11].

About 50% of women with HSDD respond to flibanserin and it may take up to 8 weeks before its effectiveness is manifested. The most common adverse events (AE) in premenopausal patients are dizziness (9.2%), sleepiness (8.3%), nausea (6.5%), and fatigue (3.7%).

Another treatment is the **bupropion**, which acts by enhancing dopamine and norepinephrine, but side effects include tremor (13.5%), agitation (9.7%), dry mouth (9.2%), constipation (8.2%), dizziness (6.1%), and nausea/vomiting (4%). However, it seems that patients with antidepressant-induced sexual dysfunction, treated with extended-release bupropion (300 mg/day) have improved sexual desire [12]. Adverse effects remain: dizziness (9%), nervousness (4%), nausea (3%), and headache (3%) [13].

On the other hand, testosterone therapy, initially approved in Europe for the treatment of *HSDD* in women in surgical menopause, is currently approved in Australia for patients with testosterone deficiency and associated symptoms, such as low sexual desire.

The fact remains that oral testosterone therapy is not recommended due to the numerous intraindividual and interindividual variables in the absorption of the treatment that can cause lipid- and cardiac-effects, as well as hepatotoxicity.

Goldstein et al. [5]—scientific research has shown, on the other hand, that transdermal testosterone therapy has positive effects for the treatment of *hypoactive sexual desire disorder* (HSDD) in both natural- and surgical-postmenopausal patients (also in combination with estrogen therapy during menopause). Four clinical studies have found that a testosterone patch of 300 μg/day (for 24 weeks) significantly improved sexual desire and the frequency of sexual intercourse in patients with HSDD in natural- and surgical-postmenopause [14].

2.6 HSDD in Men

There is not much information on hypoactive desire in men, even though the increasing number of requests for therapy from patients with HSDD seems to be on the rise. This results in the need on the part of clinicians for universal guidelines for the anamnestic and therapeutic approach.

The study by Leonard DeRogatis et al. [15] involved approximately 200 patients recruited, excluding men with erectile dysfunction, serum testosterone <300 ng/dL or depression. The following questionnaires were administered: the *Sexual Desire Inventory* (SDI), the *Male Desire Scale* (MDS), the *Sexual Concerns*

Inventory-Male (SCI-M), the *Sexual Desire Relationship Distress Scale* (SDRDS), in addition to the *University of California, Los Angeles* (UCLA) psychosexual diary. Based on a brief structured interview, the diagnosis, according to the **DSM-IV-TR** criteria for hypoactive sexual desire disorder (**HSDD**), identified a population of men with characteristics similar to patients without HSDD in terms of age, serum testosterone levels, concomitant diseases, and drug use, but distinct in their experience of sexual desire and discomfort associated with low desire.

The study by Eusebio Rubio-Aurioles et al. [16] reviewed the relevant evidence-based literature and published guidelines.

From here, the proposal of a new classification scheme: LSD/I is proposed as a generic term for which *hypoactive sexual desire disorder* (HSDD) is only a subtype. The following standard operating procedures are described: (i) detection of LSD/I: screening for LSD/I, screening for LSD/I in patients with other sexual dysfunctions; (ii) diagnosis and assessment of etiology: diagnostic criteria for LSD/I, assessment of depression status, assessment of relationship status, assessment of endocrine status, diagnostic criteria for HSDD in men; (iii) treatment of LSD/I secondary to low testosterone, treatment of LSD/I secondary to high prolactin, treatment of LSD/I secondary to other endocrine disorders, treatment of LSD/I secondary to depressive illness and/or anxiety disorders, treatment of LSD/I secondary to relational conflict, and treatment of HSDD. This would imply exclusively pharmacological therapy.

Evaluating the diagnostic criteria of the DSM, the study by Lori A. Brottoat et al. [17] examined the prevalence and correlations of low desire in men, as well as qualitative and quantitative research on the experience of sexual desire in men and women. The literature search was conducted through Medline, PubMed, and PsychInfo. The dilemma arises whether *desire and arousal can be reliably differentiated in men, and whether parallels can be drawn with the literature on women.* Finally, it proposes three options for the diagnosis of low desire in men for the DSM-5.

Option 1 proposes that the name and criteria of the *DSM-IV-TR* be retained for men in the *DSM-5*.

Option 2 proposes that the recently proposed criteria for the *Disorder of Interest/Arousal* in women be adopted also for men, which would result in a gender-neutral category. Option 3 proposes that the criteria for the *Disorder of Interest/Arousal* be applied also to men, with a slight modification regarding the physical genital changes that would seem to be excluded from the *DSM-5* criteria.

Hypoactive sexual desire disorder (HSDD) in men, characterized by chronically low sexual desire, seems associated with poor sexual well-being, such as less sexual satisfaction and greater sexual discomfort. Moreover, despite low desire, patients with HSDD often report desiring sexual intimacy and validation within their lives or sexual relationships. Studies applying self-determination theory to sexual relationships show that adopting more autonomous motivations (e.g., engaging in sex for intrinsic pleasure) and less controlled motivations (e.g., engaging in sex for an external reward or consequence) to engage in sex is associated with greater sexual well-being for both members of the couple. Since autonomous motivation in relationships is associated with intimacy and sexual satisfaction and less sexual discomfort, having sex for autonomous reasons *may allow men with HSDD and their partners to feel more sexually intimate despite their lower sexual desire, while having sex for controlled reasons may hinder intimacy, sexual satisfaction, and increase sexual discomfort.* In the cross-sectional study by McClung E et al. [18], sexual motivations and satisfaction or sexual discomfort for men with HSDD and their partners were examined in 64 couples.

Men with HSDD who had sex for *more autonomous reasons* reported greater sexual satisfaction, and both partners reported greater intimacy. Men with HSDD who conducted sex focused on the "*here and now*" experienced less sexual satisfaction, and both partners reported greater restlessness.

Clinical practice has often shown that sexual fantasies during sexual intercourse have proven to be a valid aid for patients with HSDD to promote greater eroticism and autonomous satisfaction, independent of the femininity of the partner.

It is essential to be able to identify hypoactive sexual desire disorder (HSDD), with its different levels of severity, and assess how the patient experiences or suffers from the problem.

The study by Cabello-Santamaría F et al. [19] analyzed the psychometric properties and factorial structure of the questionnaire **Sexual Desire and Aversion (DESEA)**, which evaluates sexual desire and interpersonal stress (relational problems) in male and female couples. A pilot study was conducted with a group of 1583 people, including 20,424 Spanish speakers, who responded to the questionnaire via an online link. The results showed that the DESEA questionnaire is a reliable and valid tool for evaluating desire and interpersonal stress in both women and men, in clinical and research contexts.

2.7 Conclusions

Research on sexual function benefits from the emergence and validation of new and improved questionnaires that integrate existing ones, such as the ***Center of Applied Psychology Female Sexual Questionnaire*** (CAPFS-Q) [20], which includes sexual relations with a partner, sexual practices, and dysfunctional aspects of sexual relations. The **DESEA** questionnaire has recently been created and adequately validated to identify hypoactive sexual desire disorder. All new questionnaires should be short and easy to administer, without neglecting the patient's history, any partners, emotions, sexual style, and quality of life of each individual. It follows that only a team effort can offer individual patients—men and women—a personalized therapeutic plan.

Finally, as of January 2022, the classification of female sexual dysfunctions according to the new 11th revision of the ***International Classification of Diseases***. Its definitive integration into practice is expected after a transition period of 5 years. The new nomenclature is based on a circular model of female sexual activity, eliminating the Cartesian-dualistic concept of separation of individual pathophysiological entities with "non-organic" and "organic" etiology. Sexual dysfunctions are evaluated as a complex interaction of psychological, interpersonal, social, cultural, physiological, and gender processes. The new 11th revision of the ***International Classification of Diseases*** has established clear criteria for symptomatology and disorder duration based on duration, frequency, and exposure to discomfort. Female sexual dysfunctions can be diagnosed regardless of etiology. The qualifier system allows the identification of etiological factors related to health conditions, psychological and mental disorders, use of psychoactive substances or drugs, lack of knowledge or experience, and relational, cultural, or gender factors [21].

References

1. Clayton AH, et al. International society for the study of women's sexual health care process for the management of hypoactive sexual desire disorder in women. Mayo Clin Proc. 2018;93(4):467–87.
2. McCabe MP, Sharlip ID, Lewis R, et al. Incidence and prevalence of sexual dysfunction in women and men: a consensus statement from the fourth international consultation on sexual medicine 2015. J Sex Med. 2016;13:144–52.
3. Parrocchia SJ, Goldstein AT, Goldstein SW, et al. Towards a more evidence-based nosology and nomenclature for female sexual dysfunctions – part II. J Sex Med. 2016;13:1888–906.
4. Goldfischer E, Clayton AH, Goldstein I, et al. Decreased sexual desire screener (DSDS) for the diagnosis of hypoactive sexual desire disorder in women. Obstet Gynecol. 2008;111:109S.
5. Goldstein I, Kim NN, Clayton AH, et al. Hypoactive sexual desire disorder: review of the expert panel of the International society for the study of women's sexual health (ISSWSH). Mayo Clinic Proc. 2017;92:114–28.
6. Clayton AH, Goldfischer ER, Goldstein I, et al. Validation of the decreased sexual desire screener (DSDS): a brief diagnostic tool for generalized acquired female hypoactive sexual desire disorder (HSDD). J Sex Med. 2009;6:730–8.
7. Brotto LA, Yule M. Asexuality: sexual orientation, paraphilia, sexual dysfunction, or none of the above? Arch Sex Behav. 2017;46:619–27.
8. Kilimnik CD, Meston CM. Role of body esteem in the sexual arousal and inhibition responses of women with and without a history of childhood sexual abuse. J Sex Med. 2016;13:1718–172.
9. Zeleke BM, Bell RJ, Billah B, et al. Hypoactive sexual desire dysfunction in older women living in community. Menopause. 2017;24:391–9.
10. Reichenpfader U, Gartlehner G, Morgan LC, et al. Sexual dysfunction associated with second-generation antidepressants in patients with major depressive disorder: results of a systematic review with network meta-analysis. Drug Saf. 2014;37:19–31.
11. Katz M, DeRogatis LR, Ackerman R, et al. BEGONIA trial investigators. Efficacy of flibanserin in women with hypoactive sexual desire disorder: results of the BEGONIA study. J Sex Med. 2013;10:1807–15.
12. Taylor MJ, Rudkin L, Bullemor-Day P, et al. Strategies for managing sexual dysfunction induced by antidepressant medication. Cochrane Database Syst Rev. 2013;2013:CD003382.
13. Kingsberg SA, Clayton AH, Pfaus JG. Female sexual response: current models, neurobiological basis and agents currently approved or under study for the treatment of hypoactive sexual desire disorder. CNS Drugs. 2015;29:915–33.
14. Simon J, Braunstein G, Nachtigall L, et al. The testosterone patch increases sexual activity and desire in women undergoing surgical menopause with hypoactive sexual desire disorder. J Clin Endocrinol Metab. 2005;90:5226–33.

15. DeRogatis L, Rosen RC, Goldstein I, Werneburg B, Kempthorne-Rawson J, Sand M. Characterization of hypoactive sexual desire disorder (HSDD) in men. J Sex Med. 2012;9(3):812–20. https://doi.org/10.1111/j.1743-6109.2011.02592.x.
16. Rubio-Aurioles E, Bivalacqua TJ. Standard operating procedures for low sexual desire in men. J Sex Med. 2013;10(1):94–107. https://doi.org/10.1111/j.1743-6109.2012.02778.x.
17. Lori AB. The DSM diagnostic criteria for hypoactive sexual desire disorder in men. J Sex Med. 2010;7(6):2015–30. https://doi.org/10.1111/j.1743-6109.2010.01860.x.
18. McClung E, Rosen NO, Dubé JP, Wang GA, Corsini-Munt S. Motivation when desire is low: associations between sexual motivation and sexual intimacy, sexual satisfaction, and sexual distress for men with hypoactive sexual desire disorder and their partners. Arch Sex Behav. 2024;53(3):1075–89. https://doi.org/10.1007/s10508-023-02752-x. Epub 2023 Dec 19. PMID: 38114871.
19. Cabello-Santamaría F, Cabello-García MA, Aragón-Vela J, Del Río FJ. Creating and validating the DESEA questionnaire for men and women. J Clin Med. 2020;9(7):2301. https://doi.org/10.3390/jcm9072301. PMID: 32698420; PMCID: PMC7408685.
20. Tirado-González S, Navarro-Sánchez A, Compañ-Rosique A, Luri-Prieto P, Rodríguez-Marín J, Van-der Hofstadt-Román CJ, Berenguer Soler M, Navarro-Cremades F, Gil-Guillén VF, Navarro Ortiz R, et al. Validation of the female sexuality questionnaire of the Center for Applied Psychology (CAPFS-Q). J Clin Med. 2021;10:2686. https://doi.org/10.3390/jcm10122686.
21. Pastor Z, Jonášová M. What has the new 11th revision of international classification of diseases classification brought in the categorization of female sexual dysfunctions? Czech Gynecol. 2022;87(6):432–9.

Hypoactive Sexual Desire Disorder in Women?

3

Abstract

Hypoactive sexual desire disorder (HSDD)/female sexual interest/arousal disorder (FSIAD) impacts the health-related quality of life (HRQoL) of women and their partners, yet existing measures fail to adequately capture relevant symptoms, emotional difficulties, the relationship with the partner, mood changes, and the couple's emotional disorders.

Keywords

Female and male sexual interest/arousal disorder · Health-related quality of life · Hypoactive sexual desire disorder · Patient-reported outcome · Psychometric

3.1 Introduction

The Sexual Interest and Desire Inventory-Female (SIDI-F) is a 13-item scale that quantifies the severity of symptoms in women diagnosed with hypoactive sexual desire disorder (HSDD). The validity of the SIDI-F as a measure of HSDD severity has been confirmed by a series of observations. Women with a clinical diagnosis of HSDD—based on the *Diagnostic and Statistical Manual of Mental Disorders* (DSM-5) [1] of HSDD had significantly lower SIDI-F scores compared to women diagnosed with female orgasmic disorder. There was a high correlation between scores on the SIDI-F and scores on the Female Sexual Function Index (FSFI) [2] as well as an interactive voice response version of the questionnaire on changes in sexual functioning (CSFQ) [3]. Conversely, there was a poor correlation between SIDI-F scores and scores on a slightly modified version of the marital adjustment scale (MAS) [4], an assessment of overall (non-sexual) relationship satisfaction.

The concept of personal distress related to sex is currently central to the diagnosis of all female sexual dysfunctions (FSD).

E. V. Longhi, *Hypoactive Sexual Desire Disorder*,
https://doi.org/10.1007/978-3-032-00659-2_3

Hypoactive sexual desire disorder (HSDD) and female sexual interest/arousal disorder (FSIAD) impact the health-related quality of life (HRQoL) for women and their partners, yet existing measures fail to adequately capture relevant concepts, such as the impact of symptoms, which are important for women with HSDD and FSIAD. In the study by Derogatis L. et al. [5], we find a slightly revised new version of the Female Sexual Distress Scale (FSDS), the FSDS-Revised (FSDS-R), to adapt the sensitivity of the questionnaire for patients suffering from hypoactive sexual desire disorder (HSDD). It was also shown that both instruments possess reliability and discriminant validity in premenopausal women with HSDD.

A methodological study was conducted in 27 centers in North America, enrolling 296 women aged between 18 and 50 years with HSDD, who reported a second female sexual dysfunction (FSD) or no FSD. Subjects completed the FSDS-R at baseline, on day 7, and on day 28, with a 30-day recall at baseline and a 7-day recall on days 7 and 28. The average total scores of FSDS, FSDS-R, and *FSDS-R* item 13, with both recall periods, were significantly higher ($P < 0.0001$) in women with FSD or HSDD compared to women without FSD, demonstrating that both tests had discriminative validity. The analysis confirmed the internal consistency of both tests.

The research on the validity of research questionnaires in this field also references the Polish study by Nowosielski K et al. [6]. In this survey, 210 women aged between 18 and 55 years were recruited. Seventy-five patients were diagnosed with hypoactive sexual desire disorder (HSDD), 31 were diagnosed with another FSD, and 104 patients were part of the control group. All subjects completed the PL-FSDS-R at baseline (day 0), day 7, and day 28. The average total PL-FSDS-R score was statistically higher in women with HSDD and other FSD compared to healthy individuals, demonstrating that the test had discriminative validity. The frequency of sexual intercourse and the quality of the relationship with the sexual partner—but not other sexual behaviors—were statistically correlated with the PL-FSDS-R score. This shows that the PL-FSDS-R is a reliable questionnaire with good psychometric and discriminative validity and can be used to measure personal distress related to sex in Polish women with *FSD*, with a cut-off score $\geq$13.

The research by Lim-Watson MZ [7], for example, traced studies on women with HSDD/FSIAD on PubMed, Embase, and PsychINFO from June 5, 1989, to September 30, 2020, with psychometric analyses only in English. The principles of the Preferred Reporting Items for Systematic Reviews and Meta-Analyses, the consensus-based standards for the selection of health measurement instruments, the risk-of-bias checklist, and other psychometric criteria were applied. Based on this research, 56 articles were evaluated, including 15 randomized controlled studies, 11 observational studies, and 30 psychometric studies.

Of the 18 measures identified, the Female Sexual Function Index (FSFI) and the Female Sexual Distress Scale—Revised (FSDS-R) were included in most studies (>50%). General health-related quality of life tools were not used in any of the clinical studies; SF-12, SF-36, and EQ-5D-5L were reported in two observational studies.

No tool received positive quality ratings in all psychometric criteria. FSFI, FSDS-R, Sexual Event Diary (SED), and Sexual Desire Relationship Distress Scale (SDRDS) were the only measures to receive a positive rating for content validity.

Therefore, reliable, and valid measures of health-related quality of life that include sexual desire and distress are still needed to provide a more systematic, comprehensive assessment of health-related quality of life and treatment benefits in women with HSDD/FSIAD. While there is a lack of uniformity in the concepts evaluated and psychometric assessment in women with HSDD/FSIAD, there are opportunities for the development of reliable, validated tools that comprehensively measure the most relevant, important concepts in women with HSDD/FSIAD.

3.2 Sexual Desire Relationship Distress Scale (SDRDS)

We cannot exclude the Sexual Desire Relationship Distress Scale (SDRDS), developed to meet the need for a patient-reported outcome (PRO) measure of their own sexual distress associated with hypoactive sexual desire disorder (HSDD). The SDRDS includes 17 items related to personal sexual distress and distress related to the relationship with the partner.

The study by Revicki DA et al. [8] evaluated the psychometric properties of the SDRDS among women with HSDD.

Two hundred sixty premenopausal and postmenopausal patients with or without sexual dysfunction completed the SDRDS, sexual activity questions, the Female Sexual Distress Scale-Revised (FSDS-R), and the desire domain of the Female Sexual Function Index (FSFI) at baseline, 2 weeks, and 4 weeks later.

Of the 260 patients, 101 reported pre- and postmenopausal HSDD, and 29 were part of the pre- and postmenopausal control groups. No differences emerged between pre- and postmenopausal women. The mean least squares SDRDS score was higher in women with HSDD compared to women without sexual dysfunction. Test-retest reliability was good, with an intraclass correlation coefficient of 0.89. SDRDS scores were strongly correlated with other measures of sexual distress and sexual function, including the desire domain items of FSDS-R and FSFI. Preliminary analyses suggested that the SDRDS was sensitive to changes in clinical status.

3.3 The Sexual Event Diary (SED) [9]

Going further in the investigation, the study by Van Nes Y et al. [9] evaluated the efficacy of drugs to be taken as needed for hypoactive sexual desire disorder (HSDD) or female sexual interest/arousal disorder (FSIAD), using a validated tool that analyzes individual sexual events under pharmacological therapy.

The psychometric evaluation was conducted on data from 10,959 sexual event diaries (SED), collected during three clinical studies on a total of 421 patients with HSDD. Cognitive debriefing interviews were conducted with 16 women with HSDD.

Several items from the initial 16-item SED showed weak validity. Thus, the 16-item SED was refined into an 11-item SED. The reliability, content, and convergent validity of the 11-item SED were confirmed. For most of the scores of the 11-item SED items, the ability to discriminate between the groups involved in the research was confirmed. Greater variation in the average score was found in those who benefited from the drug compared to patients without pharmacological therapy. The 11-item SED thus proved to be a reliable, valid, and responsive tool, suitable for use in evaluating the effects of on-demand drugs in women with HSDDFSIAD.

Among the strengths of the sexual event diary is the validation of the SED, performed on data from about 11,000 sexual events collected as part of a drug development program for HSDD and FSIAD. This amount of data provides very solid results when correlated with the use of drugs for HSDD and FSIAD, but caution is needed if generalizing the validity of the SED to other research areas, such as recreational drug use and risky sexual behaviors, because such information was not mentioned in the study in question.

3.4 Changes in Sexual Functioning Questionnaire (CSFQ)

The Changes in Sexual Functioning Questionnaire (CSFQ) is a 36-item clinical and research tool that identifies five scales of sexual functioning. The study by Keller A. et al. [10] documents the internal consistency and factorial structure of a 14-item version of the CSFQ (CSFQ-14), which produces scores for three scales corresponding to the phases of the sexual response cycle (desire, arousal, and orgasm), as well as the five scales of the original CSFQ. Factorial analysis confirms the construct validity of CSFQ-14 as a global measure of sexual dysfunction. CSFQ-14 and the individual scales show strong internal reliability.

A different application of this tool is provided by the multicenter study by Garcia-Portilla MP [11], which applied it to Spanish patients with mental disorders.

Eighty-nine patients with schizophrenia and 82 with bipolar disorder were evaluated using CSFQ-14, the Visual Analogue Scale for Sexual Functioning Satisfaction (VAS-SFS), and the Clinical Global Impression-Severity scale for mental disorders (CGI-S) and for sexual dysfunction (CGI-SSD).

CSFQ-14 was able to discriminate between patients with absent, mild, moderate, and severe sexual dysfunction according to CGI-SDS scores, both in males ($P < 0.001$) and females ($P < 0.001$). In males, the area under the curve (AUC) was 0.833, and a cutoff point of 49 provided a sensitivity of 92.9% and a specificity of 59.5%. In females, the AUC was 0.834, and a cutoff point of 43 provided a sensitivity of 91.9% and a specificity of 62.5%.

It should be added to this data that HSDD also affects the relatives of schizophrenic patients, in addition to depression, insomnia, and panic attacks [12].

Some validated tools are the Perceived Family Burden Scale (PFBS), the Involvement Evaluation Questionnaire (IEQ), and the Experience of Caregiving Inventory (ECI).

The development of a self-administered questionnaire to assess the subjective quality of life related to health in caregivers of schizophrenic patients seems more than necessary. The tool should be developed from the caregiver's perspective and derived from qualitative interviews with the relatives of patients suffering from schizophrenia. Its reactivity should be documented before inclusion in clinical studies or in the evaluation of psychoeducational programs.

The Changes in Sexual Functioning Questionnaire (CSFQ) is also a structured questionnaire or interview designed to measure the effects related to diseases and drugs on sexual functioning. Individuals from clinical and non-clinical samples completed the CSFQ in the study by Kleyton AH et al. [13]. The sample groups were compared on the average scores of the CSFQ and its subscales. Comparative results indicate that psychiatric patients diagnosed with a mood disorder have significantly lower sexual functioning compared to nonpsychiatric outpatients, medical students, and psychiatry residents combined. The CSFQ is a useful measure to systematically assess the effects related to diseases or drugs on sexual functioning.

3.5 Conclusions

Hypoactive Sexual Desire Disorder (HSDD) and Sexual Aversion Disorder (SAD) are groups of underdiagnosed disorders that affect men and women. Despite their prevalence, these two disorders are often not addressed by healthcare providers and patients due to their private and embarrassing nature. Specialists often feel inadequate and uncomfortable in deciding appropriate treatment. Using the sexual response cycle as a model of human physiological changes during sexual stimulation and the *Diagnostic and Statistical Manual of Mental Disorders, fourth edition*, along with many validated questionnaires, it is possible to trace the co-causes of HSDD. The National Health and Social Life Survey found that 32% of women, and 15% of men, had no sexual interest for several months in the last year. The patients were aged between 18 and 59 years [14].

The proposed etiology of HSDD influences how it is subtyped (generalized or situational, lifelong or acquired). For example, lifelong HSDD may be due to problems with sexual identity—gender identity, orientation, or paraphilia—or stagnation in sexual growth—overly conservative context, developmental anomalies, or abuse. Conversely, difficulties in a new sexual relationship can lead to an acquired or situational subtype of HSDD. Although it is theoretically possible to have no etiology, all appropriate avenues should be explored, including whether the patient has been truthful in responses to questions about sexuality and whether the patient is aware of having a sexual disorder.

References

1. American Psychiatric Association, editor. Diagnostic and statistical manual of mental disorders. 4th ed. Washington, DC: American Psychiatric Association; 2000.
2. Rosen RC. Prevalence and risk factors of sexual dysfunction in men and women. Curr Psychiatry Rep. 2000;3:189–95.
3. Clayton AH, McGarvey EL, Clavet GJ. The changes in sexual functioning questionnaire (CSFQ): development, reliability, and validity. Psychopharmacol Bull. 1997;33:731–45.

4. Locke HJ, Wallace KM. Locke-Wallace marital adjustment scale and prediction test: their reliability and validity. Marriage Fam Living. 1959;2:251–5.
5. Derogatis L, Clayton A, Lewis-D'Agostino D, Wunderlich G, Fu Y. Validation of the female sexual distress scale-revised for assessing distress in women with hypoactive sexual desire disorder. J Sex Med. 2008;5(2):357–64. https://doi.org/10.1111/j.1743-6109.2007.00672.x. Epub 2007 Nov 27. PMID: 18042215.
6. Nowosielski K, Wróbel B, Sioma-Markowska U, Poręba R. Sexual dysfunction and distress–development of a Polish version of the female Sexual Distress Scale-Revised. J Sex Med. 2013;10(5):1304–12. https://doi.org/10.1111/jsm.12112. Epub 2013 Feb 27. PMID: 23444946.
7. Lim-Watson MZ, Hays RD, Kingsberg S, Kallich JD, Murimi-Worstell IB. A systematic literature review of health-related quality of life measures for women with hypoactive sexual desire disorder and female sexual interest/arousal disorder. Sex Med Rev. 2022;10(1):23–41.
8. Revicki DA, Margolis MK, Fisher W, Rosen RC, Kuppermann M, Hanes V, Sand M. Evaluation of the sexual desire relationship distress scale (SDRDS) in women with hypoactive sexual desire disorder. J Sex Med. 2012;9(5):1344–54.
9. Van Nes Y, Bloemers J, van der Heijden PGM, van Rooij K, Gerritsen J, Kessels R, DeRogatis L, Tuiten A. The sexual event diary (SED): development and validation of a standardized questionnaire for assessing female sexual functioning during discrete sexual events. J Sex Med. 2017;14:1438.
10. Keller A, McGarvey EL, Clayton AH. Reliability and construct validity of the changes in sexual functioning questionnaire short-form (CSFQ-14). J Sex Marital Ther. 2006;32(1):43–52.
11. Garcia-Portilla MP, Saiz PA, Fonseca E, Al-Halabi S, Bobes-Bascaran MT, Arrojo M, Benabarre A, Goikolea JM, Sanchez E, Sarramea F, Bobes J. Psychometric properties of the Spanish version of the changes in sexual functioning questionnaire short-form (CSFQ-14) in patients with severe mental disorders. J Sex Med. 2011;8(5):1371–82. https://doi.org/10.1111/j.1743-6109.2010.02043.x. Epub 2010 Oct 4. PMID: 20946156.
12. Reine G, Lancon C, Simeoni MC, Duplan S, Auquier P. Caregiver burden in relatives of persons with schizophrenia: an overview of measure instruments. Encephale. 2003;29(2):137–47. French. PMID: 14567165.
13. Clayton AH, McGarvey EL, Clavet GJ, Piazza L. Comparison of sexual functioning in clinical and nonclinical populations using the changes in sexual functioning questionnaire (CSFQ). Psychopharmacol Bull. 1997;33(4):747–53. PMID: 9493487.
14. Levine SB, editor. Sexual disorders. In Tasman A, Kay J, Lieberman J. Psychiatry, 2nd edition. Hoboken: Wiley; 2003.

Hypoactive Sexual Desire Disorder in Men

4

Abstract

Hypoactive sexual desire disorder (HSDD), which emerged in the late 1970s with the rise of sexual therapy (listed in the *Diagnostic and Statistical Manual of Mental Disorders*), has gained increasing attention—promotion and a reaction of criticism—with the rise of the pharmaceutical industry's influence in sexual research. The relationship of these categories has often been noted but largely unexplored, especially in the context of ***men's HSDD***. So far, research has focused more on female HSDD. Even the study by Segraves, K. B et al. (J Sex Marital Ther 17:55–58, 1991), involving 906 subjects (studied in a multisite pharmaceutical study) with a primary diagnosis of HSDD, found that: HSDD was much more common in females than in male subjects. Males diagnosed with HSDD were significantly older. Approximately 40% of subjects with a primary diagnosis of HSDD had a secondary diagnosis of arousal or orgasm disorders. But today, research has found otherwise.

Keywords

Hypoactive sexual desire disorder · Sexual interest · Sexual desire · DSM diagnostic criteria · Self-determination theory · Sexual discomfort · Sexual motivation · Sexual satisfaction · Patient-reported outcomes · Maintenance therapy with methadone · Smoking · Relationship · Post-traumatic stress disorder · Neurobiology · Neuroendocrinology

4.1 Introduction

Through many studies and different measures, men have been shown to have more frequent and intense sexual desires than women, as evidenced by spontaneous thoughts about sex, the frequency and variety of sexual fantasies, the desired frequency of intercourse, the desired number of partners, masturbation, liking for

E. V. Longhi, *Hypoactive Sexual Desire Disorder*,
https://doi.org/10.1007/978-3-032-00659-2_4

various sexual practices, willingness to give up sex, initiating or refusing sex, making sacrifices for sex, and other measures [1].

In 2004–2005, for example, a sample of 7001 men aged 18 or older was recruited from gay-oriented sexual networking, chat, and news sites. Patients reported having had male sexual partners throughout their lives and having had oral or anal sex with a male partner in their most recent encounter in the past year.

Seven questions about SD symptoms that occurred in the past 12 months concerned low sexual desire, erection problems, inability to achieve orgasm, performance anxiety, premature ejaculation, pain during sex, and unenjoyable sex.

Self-reported symptoms of SD appeared high. Overall, 79% of men reported one or more symptoms of SD in the past year, including ***low sexual desire, erection problems, and performance anxiety, being the most common***.

The LCA identified four distinct underlying patterns of sexual functioning [2].

Absent or low SD, erection problems or performance anxiety, low desire or pleasure, and high SD or sexual pain. High SD or sexual pain was distinguished from the other patterns based on the use of club drugs and the use of prescription and nonprescription erectile dysfunction drugs before sexual intercourse in the past year. In addition, men associated with the high SD or sexual pain group were younger, single, more likely to have poor mental and physical health, and more likely to have been diagnosed with a sexually transmitted infection in the past year compared to men in the no or low DS group.

The fact remains that male sexual problems are much more common than thought, particularly hypoactive sexual desire disorder. However, clinical attention to male HSDD still appears limited [3].

The *Good-Enough Sex* model, for example, could provide physicians with crucial elements to address this pathology, promoting the positive value of sex, acceptance of realistic expectations, promotion of sexual flexibility, and variable quality of intimacy.

4.2 Diagnostic Criteria

The study by Lori A. Brotto et al. [4] conducted a literature search on *Medline, PubMed, and PsychInfo* to identify any publications on low desire in men.

The dilemma of whether desire and arousal can be reliably differentiated in men is discussed, and parallels are drawn with the literature on women. Finally, three options for the diagnosis of low desire in men for the DSM-5 are considered.

Option 1 proposes that the name and criteria of the DSM-IV-TR be retained for men in the DSM-5.

Option 2 proposes that the recently proposed criteria for Sexual Interest/Arousal Disorder in women be adopted also for men, which would result in a gender-neutral category.

Option 3 proposes that the criteria for Sexual Interest/Arousal Disorder be applied also to men, with a small modification to one criterion (i.e., that absent or reduced genital and non-genital physical changes are not included as a criterion); this diagnosis would then only be applied to men.

However, ***despite low desire, men with HSDD often report desiring sexual intimacy and validation within their sexual lives and relationships***. Studies applying self-determination theory to sexual relationships show that adopting more autonomous motivations (for example, engaging in sex for its intrinsic pleasure) and less controlled motivations (for example, engaging in sex for an external reward or consequence) for engaging in sex is associated with greater sexual well-being for both members of the couple. Since autonomous motivation in relationships is associated with intimacy, sexual satisfaction, and less sexual distress, having sex for autonomous reasons may allow men with HSDD and their partners to feel more sexually intimate despite their lower sexual desire, *while having sex for controlled reasons may hinder intimacy, sexual satisfaction, and increase sexual distress.*

In the study by McClung E et al. [5], the associations between types of sexual motivation and sexual intimacy, sexual satisfaction, and sexual distress for men with HSDD and their partners ($n = 64$ couples) were examined. Men with HSDD who reported having sex for more autonomous reasons reported greater sexual satisfaction, and both partners reported greater sexual intimacy. Men with HSDD who had sex for more controlled reasons had partners who experienced less intimacy and sexual satisfaction, and both partners were more sexually stressed. Promoting autonomous sexual motivation and reducing controlled motivation may help couples dealing with HSDD to feel closer in their relationship, more sexually satisfied, and less sexually stressed.

The study by Leonard DeRogatis [6] provided a first comprehensive characterization of men diagnosed with HSDD *Diagnostic and Statistical Manual of Mental Disorders*, fourth edition, text revision (DSM-IV-TR), using consolidated patient-reported outcomes (PRO) and new PROs developed in line with the guidelines of the U.S. Food and Drug Administration (FDA).

In summary, he recruited **200** men with or without symptoms of low sexual desire and related distress. Men with erectile dysfunction, serum testosterone <300 ng/dL, or depression were excluded. The men completed evaluations of sexual desire and sex-related distress and underwent structured clinical interviews for the diagnosis of HSDD.

The primary endpoints were the scores of the Sexual Desire Inventory (SDI), the Male Desire Scale (MDS), the Sexual Concerns Inventory–Male (SCI-M), and the Sexual Desire Relationship Distress Scale (SDRDS) on day 28, and the University of California, Los Angeles (UCLA) psychosexual diary scores on days 21–27.

The results showed that there were no clinically relevant differences in terms of age, serum testosterone, depressive symptoms, erectile function, concomitant diseases, or use of medications between men with HSDD ($N = 109$) and men without HSDD ($N = 91$). However, there were ***clinically significant differences between men with and without HSDD in sexual desire*** and in sex-related distress, according to the SCI-M score, and in the score of the UCLA Psychosexual Diary sexual activity domain.

Based on a brief structured interview, the diagnosis (according to DSM-IV-TR criteria) for HSDD identified a population of men comparable to men without HSDD in terms of age, serum testosterone, concomitant disease, and use of medications, but distinct in their experience of sexual desire and distress associated with low desire.

4.3 HSDD and Opioid Use

Methadone maintenance therapy (MMT) was introduced in 2005, and this medication-assisted therapy (MAT) program has significantly reduced the spread of intravenously transmitted diseases such as human immunodeficiency virus (HIV), hepatitis B, and hepatitis C. Sexual dysfunction related to the use of methadone in men is attributed to a reduction in gonadotropin-releasing hormone (GnRH) and luteinizing hormone (LH), leading to reduced plasma levels of testosterone [7]. One meta-analysis has reported that the prevalence of sexual dysfunction in this patient group was 52% (95% confidence interval [CI], 0.4–0.6), and hypoactive sexual desire and low libido were the most common [8]. Many previous studies have used the International Index of Erectile Function 15 (IIEF-15) to assess low sexual desire among MMT men for ease of completion. However, the IIEF-15 appears primarily a validated tool to measure erectile dysfunction in men rather than orgasmic function or sexual desire. Therefore, this scale may not be the most suitable tool to assess sexual desire [9]. Evidence of the relationship between low sexual desire and quality of life (QOL) among men undergoing MMT remains scant. A recent cross-sectional study identified that men undergoing MAT who scored low in the sexual desire domain of the IIEF-15 reported a lower quality of life, especially in their social relationships, compared to those who underwent buprenorphine maintenance treatment [10]. Furthermore, patients with low libido reported that the quality of their sexual relationships with their partners was strongly conditioned [11]. The study by Yee A et al. [8] included male subjects aged 18 years or older with a history of opioid dependence according to the *Diagnostic and Statistical Manual*, fourth Edition (DSM-IV), and those who had been undergoing methadone-assisted treatment for at least 2 months before the interview. Patients with unstable medical or psychiatric diseases, those concurrently taking antiviral drugs for viral hepatitis or HIV, androgen replacement therapy, or type 5 phosphodiesterase inhibitors, as well as those using psychotropic drugs other than methadone, were excluded. The study was completed by 183 male patients undergoing MMT. The patients had an average age of 43.8 years, were predominantly male, married, had a secondary level of education, and full-time employment. They did not have a family history of substance abuse. The average dose of methadone taken was 72.5 mg for an average duration of 49.9 months. Additionally, 36.6% tested positive for hepatitis C, 4.4% for hepatitis B, and 2.2% had other medical conditions such as hypertension, diabetes mellitus, and dyslipidemia. This study reported that 32.8% of male patients undergoing MMT, about 60, had low desire for sexual desire (DSD) and sexual satisfaction desire (SSD); 26.8%, about 40 patients, showed normal DSD but low SSD; and

9.8%, about 18 patients, had low DSD but normal SSD. Furthermore, 32.8% of patients undergoing MMT were diagnosed with low sexual desire [12]. It was also observed that MMT patients have a significantly higher smoking rate compared to the general population. A systematic review reported that smoking rates for MMT patients ranged from 73.5% to 94.0% [13]. However, evidence regarding the effects of smoking on sexual desire in this patient group remains limited. In fact, an increase in the frequency and number of cigarettes smoked daily was associated with low sexual desire. The higher prevalence of smoking in MMT patients translates into a significantly increased risk of morbidity and mortality related to tobacco use.

4.3.1 Male HSDD and Brain Functions

Clinical research has advanced further. The primary objective was to identify, in patients with HSDD, the brain regions where functional disturbances disrupt the regulation of sexual motivation [14]. Positron emission tomography was used to compare seven male patients with HSDD with eight healthy men by examining their regional cerebral blood flow responses to graded-intensity visual sexual stimuli (VSS). Statistical parametric mapping was used to identify brain regions that demonstrated differential activation (or deactivation) in the groups. While in control subjects the medial orbitofrontal cortex showed a deactivation in response to VSS, patients with HSDD exhibited abnormally maintained activity in this region, which has been implicated in the inhibitory control of motivated behavior. Conversely, the inverse pattern—activation in control subjects and deactivation or unchanged activity in patients—was observed in the secondary somatosensory cortex and **in the inferior parietal lobules**, regions that mediate emotional and motor imagination processes, as well as in areas of the anterior **cingulate gyrus** and frontal lobes involved in premotor processes.

Regarding clinical studies, HSDD has been reported as the most frequent cause of consultation among sexual disorders. In a pharmacological therapy study for sexual dysfunctions, 65% of patients received a primary diagnosis of HSDD. However, little is yet known about the etiology of HSDD, which is considered the most difficult to treat among psychosexual disorders.

With regard to comorbidity, male patients with a DSM-III diagnosis of inhibited sexual desire without current associated Axis I disorder had high lifetime prevalence rates of affective disorder compared to controls without sexual disorders. Similarly, increases in scores on the depression scale of the Symptom Checklist-90-R have been reported in patients with HSDD. ***HSDD is often concomitant with erectile dysfunction. In a sample of 113 males with HSDD, 53 (47%) had erectile impairment***. Although it is likely that erectile dysfunction is a consequence of HSDD, it has also been proposed that the lack of sexual pleasure and performance anxiety due to erectile dysfunction may decrease sexual desire.

Relationship problems have also been considered as contributing factors to HSDD, emphasizing that these patients unconsciously downregulate their sexual desires by selectively focusing on characteristics they judge to be negative in their partners.

Furthermore, since it can be shown which brain regions activate or deactivate in response to sexual stimuli, functional brain imaging techniques are likely to be useful for determining:

1. *Whether the pathophysiological mechanism is the essential element of HSDD.*
2. *Whether there is an abnormal functioning of the brain regions that control sexual motivation and, more specifically.*
3. *Whether HSDD derives from an intrinsically low level.*
4. *From an inhibition of sexual motivation from both mechanisms.*

The study by Janssen E et al. [15] focused on developing and initially validating a questionnaire that measures the propensity for sexual inhibition and excitation in men: the ***Sexual Inhibition Sexual Excitation Scales (SIS/SES)***. The basic theoretical model postulates that sexual response and associated behavior depend on dual control mechanisms, involving excitatory and inhibitory neurophysiological systems. The scales, along with their discriminant and convergent validity and test-retest reliability, are described.

In a sample of 408 sexually functional men (average age = 22.8 years), factor analyses identified three higher-level factors: two related to sexual inhibition and one to sexual excitation. Multigroup confirmatory factor analyses revealed that the factorial structure provided an acceptable fit to the data obtained in a second ($N = 459$; average age = 20.9 years) and third ($N = 313$; average age = 46.2 years) sample of men, with similar distributions and relationships with other measures.

4.3.2 HSDD in the Pathology of "Huntington's Disease"

There are only a few studies in the literature on sexuality in Huntington's disease that conclude up to 85% of men and up to 75% of women experience high levels of sexual problems, most of which present prevalent symptoms of a *hypoactive sexual disorder*, but an increase in sexual interest and paraphilia have also been found [16]. There is no evidence that sexual dysfunction is primarily a specific symptom of HD and may be associated with the specific brain lesion itself or if it is primarily related to the psychosocial factors caused by the constant worsening of the disease. Further studies should focus on asymptomatic patients to explore sexual changes that precede neurological and motor symptoms and should incorporate partners to objectify distinctive sexual characteristics. Investigations into the context of sexual dysfunction with depression, irritability, and dementia symptoms are needed to better understand the reasons for sexual changes in HD. Treatment options for HD patients with sexual disorders are reported only sporadically, guidelines can only be obtained from non-HD patients and further research is needed.

4.4 HSDD and Post-traumatic Stress Disorder (PTSD) [17]

HSDD is a common clinical disorder in survivors of post-traumatic stress disorder (PTSD) trauma. As there are biological parallels in the neuroendocrine processes underlying both PTSD and sexual behavior, the study by Lehrner A et al. [18] conducted an exploratory investigation into the relationship between PTSD and neuroendocrine indicators associated with sexual dysfunction in armed service veterans. Major depressive disorder, which is highly comorbid with PTSD and sexual dysfunction, was also evaluated. In veterans with PTSD, sexual problems were associated with plasma dehydroepiandrosterone (DHEA) and cortisol, urinary catecholamines, and glucocorticoid sensitivity, even when controlling for the effects of comorbid depression. In a subsample analysis, testosterone levels did not distinguish PTSD or sexual dysfunction, suggesting that the sexual problems reported by veterans in this sample were not the result of an organic disorder. PTSD predicted higher levels of dihydrotestosterone (DHT), which were associated with sexual problems. Moreover, since the onset of conflicts in Iraq and Afghanistan, over two million Americans have served in war. More than half of the 1.5 million who are eligible for healthcare from the Department of Veterans Affairs (VA) have enrolled upon returning from their missions. Over half of these veterans have received mental health diagnoses, the most common of which is post-traumatic stress disorder (PTSD). PTSD has been associated with multiple physical health disorders in Operation Iraqi Freedom/Operation Enduring Freedom (OIF/OEF) and previous era veterans. National representative samples and clinical studies have used anonymous and confidential self-assessment questionnaires to determine the prevalence of sexual dysfunction. For men under 35, estimates of erectile dysfunction based on direct questions have ranged from 2% to 14% [19], and a prevalence of (HSDD) of 5.5% has been found. Furthermore, veterans who have received a PTSD diagnosis had a prevalence of HSDD greater than 10%, which increased to nearly 13% among those prescribed psychiatric medications. Selective serotonin reuptake inhibitors (SSRIs) are the most frequently prescribed drugs nationwide and are approved by the U.S. Food and Drug Administration (FDA) for PTSD and depression [20]. SSRIs are associated with ejaculatory dysfunction, such as delayed ejaculation, inability to ejaculate, and absent or delayed orgasm [21]. Before starting psychiatric pharmacological therapy, an evaluation of baseline sexual function can help quantify side effects should they occur.

4.4.1 Cystectomy and HSDD

Cystectomy is a urological surgical procedure indicated for a range of conditions, including muscle-invasive bladder cancer, recurrent and refractory noninvasive bladder tumors, radiation injuries, and severe end-stage bladder dysfunction. Of the 73,000 men and women diagnosed with bladder cancer each year, about 25% present with invasive or advanced-stage disease and can be managed with cystectomy. In men, cystectomy involves removal of the bladder, prostate, and seminal vesicles.

In women, cystectomy typically includes removal of the uterus, ovaries, fallopian tubes, cervix, and the anterior portion of the vagina, although in some cases vaginal and organ-sparing procedures are performed. Urinary diversion is performed alongside cystectomy to redirect urine out of the body and is an ancillary part of the surgical procedure [22]. In the United States, between 8000 and 10,000 cystectomies and urinary diversions are performed each year. As with other pelvic surgical procedures, cystectomy is associated with significant changes in sexual function for both men and women. For example, erectile dysfunction can affect up to 80% of men after cystectomy and urinary diversion; the same percentage applies for HSDD. Body alterations associated with urinary diversion and the resulting changes in body image, emotional, and psychological responses of both patients and their partners can compromise sexuality and sexual satisfaction and strain intimate relationships.

Health-related quality of life (HRQOL) questionnaires like the FACT-B ask for information about interest in sex, while the Brief Sexual Function Inventory (BCI) goes further, asking for information about desire, arousal, sensation, and orgasm. The absence of orgasms (anorgasmia), changes in intensity, climacteric, and pain with orgasm (dysorgasmia) can be significant problems in this population, as they are among men treated with prostatectomy for prostate cancer. Hypogonadism may be another influencing factor that has been incompletely studied among patients undergoing cystectomy [23]. Symptomatic hypogonadism affects about 5.6% of men between the ages of 30 and 79 and increases with age; 18.5% of men over age 60 have experienced symptomatic hypogonadism [24].

4.4.2 The Psyche

In addition to daily concerns about recurrence and disease status, bladder cancer patients treated with cystectomy and urinary diversion may also face additional stress factors related to the consequences of surgery, such as an altered body image. The presence and adaptation to a urinary stoma, for example, can not only cause body image issues but also be a source of further stress and/or depression.

Even among patients with a neobladder, who do not undergo the same degree of body alteration as patients with an ileal conduit, poor urine control and incontinence can be significant stress factors that may limit interest in sexual activity. While neobladders have been widely adopted to avoid external body changes (the presence of a stoma) and restore voluntary urinary function after bladder removal, their ability to preserve or improve body image has not been clearly demonstrated.

The psychosexual consequences, including hypoactive sexual desire disorder (HSDD), of aggressive surgeries are often studied, though without the inclusion of a preliminary sexual history to compare the characteristics of sexual activity prior to the cancer diagnosis.

The comparison could provide significant information on the co-causes of each individual patient's HSDD and assess the extent of physiological, psychological, and relational precedence if compromised over time.

4.5 Inflammatory Bowel Diseases and HSDD

Inflammatory bowel diseases (IBD) are a group of idiopathic, chronic, inflammatory intestinal diseases that are divided into two main types: **ulcerative colitis (UC) and Crohn's disease (CD)** [25]. *IBD is usually diagnosed in young individuals between the ages of 15 and 30.* Commonly [26], it is more frequent in Western countries than in other areas of the world, with a prevalence exceeding 0.3% and affecting over 3.5 million individuals, according to the most recent statistics available [27].

As a chronic, permanent disorder, IBD can impact health in various ways, such as abdominal pain, diarrhea, and fatigue during the active phase of IBD. Moreover, many studies have shown that IBD can cause severe depression and decline in health-related and sexual quality of life, including HSDD.

Several studies in recent years have highlighted that sexual problems are more common among patients with IBD compared to the general population of similar age [28]. The proportion of sexual dysfunction, reported by Knowles et al. and Mahmood et al. [29, 30], varies between 44–53.9% and 40–66% in male and female patients, respectively. Furthermore, there is evidence indicating that IBD does not influence every specific aspect of sexual function [31].

A literature search was conducted using the PubMed, Web of Science, and EMBASE databases, with restrictions to the English language and the publication period between January 1, 1990, and September 1, 2020. The main search terms were sexual function, sexual dysfunction, sexual desire disorders, *sexual arousal disorders*, erectile dysfunction, premature ejaculation, orgasm disorders, sexual pain disorders, IBD, *ulcerative colon*, and *Crohn's disease*.

Sexual function was measured by any existing and validated scale, such as the *International Index of Erectile Function* (IIEF), the *Female Sexual Function Index* (FSFI), the *Brief Index of Sexual Functioning in Women* (BISF-W), the *Arizona Sexual Experience Scale* (ASEX), and the Sexual Quality of Life Questionnaire (SQoL) [32].

Sexual health [33] is a vital issue in IBD, as IBD usually affects teenagers or younger individuals who are in the self-development and reproduction phase. A recent study of 69 men who had just been diagnosed with IBD concluded that 39% had overall SD and 94% suffered from ED and HSDD [34]. A previous study found that 44% of men felt severely sexually compromised due to IBD, mainly in those with active disease [35]. Moreover, in men with IBD, a decrease in sexual desire was more frequent compared to the general population. In agreement with this point, Marín et al. [36] showed a third of men felt that desire and sexual satisfaction worsened after the diagnosis of IBD.

As for the duration of the disease and SD, the results are controversial. Muller et al. reported that patients of both sexes with a long duration of the disease (>3 years) were 2.59 times more likely to have a decrease in libido or a total absence ($p = 0.053$) [37]. However, a previous study showed that a disease duration >10 years was not a determining factor of low sexual function in women with IBD, unlike the presence of depression.

The evaluation of disease activity: the heterogeneity among studies is primarily based on clinical scales. One study reported an association between sexual dysfunction (SD) and clinical activity of the disease—*Crohn's Disease Activity Index* (CDAI) for Crohn's disease, *Colitis Activity Index* (CAI) for ulcerative colitis—in men with inflammatory bowel disease (IBD). On the other hand, a study conducted on 168 women and 119 men with IBD showed that patients with active disease had significantly lower scores on hypoactive sexual desire disorder (HSDD) compared to patients in remission; however, the association between clinical activity and SD was explained by depression [35].

Fatigue [38] is a common symptom in IBD and is present in up to 50% of patients at the time of diagnosis. Although its origin is multifactorial, it has been correlated, among other factors, to the inflammatory activity of the disease [39]. Furthermore, fatigue has been reported in up to 40% of patients in clinical remission based on symptom scales—*Harvey-Bradshaw Index* (HBI) in Crohn's disease and *CAI* in ulcerative colitis) [40].

Interestingly, a study by Marín et al. [36] on patients with IBD and SD found that fatigue was the main symptom reported by patients as a determining factor in the deterioration of their sexual activity after diagnosis of IBD.

Currently, there are no recommendations or clinical guidelines for the treatment of SD in patients with IBD. Although the impact of IBD on sexual function is a frequent concern in patients, physicians rarely consider this issue when discussing therapeutic goals with patients.

In a study by Marin et al., 64% of women and nearly half of the men interviewed wanted to receive information about the impact that IBD would have on their intimacy and sexuality at the time of diagnosis—mainly from an IBD specialist [41]. This study conducted a postal survey on IBD patients aged between 25 and 65 years from two tertiary centers. Patients were asked to provide data on a control of the same sex and age without IBD. The questionnaire evaluated the patient's perception of the impact of IBD on their own sexuality and also allowed the calculation of the *Erectile Function International Index or the Female Sexual Function Index*.

For the final analysis, a total of 355 patients and 200 in the control group were available. Both groups were comparable, except for a higher percentage of individuals who had been treated for depression among the patients. Half of the women and a third of the men felt that both sexual desire and satisfaction had worsened after diagnosis of IBD. Compared to the control group, both men and women with IBD showed significantly lower scores on the sexual function indices.

4.5.1 Conclusions

Given the complexity of HSDD especially in men, research has sought to validate a questionnaire that measures sexual function and desire: *The SAD–MEN*, especially in Asian diabetic patients. Although erectile dysfunction is very common among men with diabetes, it is closely related to other sexual disorders such as premature ejaculation and libido issues [42]. *The SAD–MEN* questionnaire is the first to assess the factors contributing to sexual dysfunction: the duration of diabetes, polytherapy, and the side effects of certain pharmacological agents, such as antidepressants, antihypertensives, antihistamines, and diuretics, as well as assessing the patient's medical background of conditions that required these drugs for treatment [43]. The strength of this study lies in the ability of *SAD–MEN* to comprehensively assess all components of sexual dysfunction. This tool is also available in English and Malay and is culturally acceptable to the multiethnic Malaysian population. However, due to the nature of the tool—self-administration—only literate participants were recruited, mostly urbanized Malaysians (97%). This new tool, developed based on Southeast Asian men, has wide application across Asia and can contribute to early diagnosis and management of sexual dysfunction to improve quality of life. From here, Western researchers could hypothesize other research questionnaires with more survey items on the variables of HSDD.

References

1. Baumeister RF, Catanese KR, Vohs KD. Is there a gender difference in strength of sex drive? Theoretical views, conceptual distinctions, and a review of relevant evidence. Pers Soc Psychol Rev. 5(3) https://doi.org/10.1207/S15327957PSPR0503_5.
2. Hirshfield S, Chiasson MA, Wagmiller RL Jr, Remien RH, Humberstone M, Scheinmann R, Grov C. Sexual dysfunction in an internet sample of U.S. men who have sex with men. J Sex Med. 2010;7(9):3104–14. https://doi.org/10.1111/j.1743-6109.2009.01636.x. PMID: 19968773; PMCID: PMC2936665
3. Metz ME, McCarthy BW. Male sexuality and couple sexual health: a case illustration. J Fam Psychother. 2010;21(3):197–212. https://doi.org/10.1080/08975353.2010.505535.
4. Brotto LA. The DSM diagnostic criteria for hypoactive sexual desire disorder in men. J Sex Med. 2010;7(6):2015–30. https://doi.org/10.1111/j.1743-6109.2010.01860.x.
5. McClung E, Rosen NO, Dubé JP, Wang GA, Corsini-Munt S. Motivation when desire is low: associations between sexual motivation and sexual intimacy, sexual satisfaction, and sexual distress for men with hypoactive sexual desire disorder and their partners. Arch Sex Behav. 2024;53(3):1075–89. https://doi.org/10.1007/s10508-023-02752-x. Epub 2023 Dec 19. PMID: 38114871.
6. DeRogatis L, Rosen RC, Goldstein I, Werneburg B, Kempthorne-Rawson J, Sand M. Characterization of hypoactive sexual desire disorder (HSDD) in men. J Sex Med. 2012;9(3):812–20. https://doi.org/10.1111/j.1743-6109.2011.02592.x.
7. Bawor M, Bami H, Dennis BB, Plater C, Worster A, Varenbut M, Anglin R. Testosterone suppression in opioid users: a systematic review and meta-analysis. Drug Alcohol Depend. 2015;149:1–9.
8. Yee A, Loh HS, Ng CG. The prevalence of sexual dysfunction among male patients undergoing methadone and buprenorphine treatments: a meta-analysis study. J Sex Med. 2014;11(1):22–32.
9. Rosen RC, Cappelleri JC, Gendrano N. The international index of erectile function (IIEF): a state-of-the-art review. Int J Impot Res. 2002;14(4):226–44.
10. Yee A, Danaee M, Loh HS, Sulaiman AH, Ng CG. Sexual dysfunction in heroin addicts: a comparison between methadone and buprenorphine maintenance treatment. PLoS One. 2016;11(1):e0147852.
11. Xia Y, Zhang D, Li X, Chen W, He Q, Jahn HJ, Ling L. Sexual dysfunction during methadone maintenance treatment and its influence on patient's life and treatment: a qualitative study in Southern China. Psychol Health Med. 2013;18(3):321–9.

12. Mitchell KR, Mercer CH, Ploubidis GB, Jones KG, Datta J, Field N, Sonnenberg P. Sexual function in Britain: findings from the third National Survey of sexual attitudes and lifestyles (Natsal-3). Lancet. 2013;382(9907):1817–29.
13. Guydish J, Passalacqua E, Tajima B, Chan M, Chun J, Bostrom A. Smoking prevalence in addiction treatment: a review. Nicotine Tob Res. 2011;13(6):401–11.
14. Stoléru S, Redouté J, Costes N, Lavenne F, Le Bars D, Dechaud H, Forest MG, Pugeat M, Cinotti L, Pujol J-F. Brain processing of visual sexual stimuli in men with hypoactive sexual desire disorder. Psychiatry Res Neuroimaging. 2003;124(2):67–86. ISSN 0925-4927, https://doi.org/10.1016/S0925-4927(03)00068-4.
15. Janssen E, Vorst H, Finn P, Bancroft J. The sexual inhibition (SIS) and sexual excitation (SES) scales: I. Measuring sexual inhibition and excitation proneness in men. J Sex Res. 2002;39(2):114–26. https://doi.org/10.1080/00224490209552130.
16. Schmidt EZ, Bonelli RM. Sexuality in Huntington's disease. Wien Med Wochenschr. 2008;158(3–4):78–83. https://doi.org/10.1007/s10354-007-0477-8.
17. Yehuda R, Lehrner A, Rosenbaum TY. PTSD and sexual dysfunction in men and women. J Sex Med. 2015;12(5):1107–19. https://doi.org/10.1111/jsm.12856. Epub 2015 Apr 6. PMID: 25847589.
18. Lehrner A, Flory JD, Bierer LM, Makotkine I, Marmar CR, Yehuda R. Sexual dysfunction and neuroendocrine correlates of posttraumatic stress disorder in combat veterans: preliminary findings. Psychoneuroendocrinology. 2016;63:271–5. https://doi.org/10.1016/j.psyneuen.2015.10.015. Epub 2015 Oct 23. PMID: 26529050.
19. Feldman HA, Goldstein I, Hatzichristou DG, Krane RJ, McKinlay JB. Impotence and its medical and psychosocial correlates: results from the Massachusetts male aging study. J Urol. 1994;151:54–61.
20. Hidalgo RB, Davidson JR. Selective serotonin reuptake inhibitors in post-traumatic stress disorder. J Psychopharmacol. 2000;14:70–6. https://doi.org/10.1177/026988110001400110.
21. Rosen RC, Lane RM, Menza M. Effects of SSRIs on sexual function: a critical review. J Clin Psychopharmacol. 1999;19:67–85.
22. Gallagher DJ, Milowsky MI. Bladder cancer. Curr Treat Options in Oncol. 2009;10:205–15. https://doi.org/10.1007/s11864-009-0112-6.
23. Matsuda T, Aptel I, Exbrayat C, Grosclaude P. Determinants of quality of life of bladder cancer survivors five years after treatment in France. Int J Urol. 2003;10:423–9. https://doi.org/10.1046/j.1442-2042.2003.00657.x.
24. Salonia A, Burnett AL, Graefen M, Hatzimouratidis K, Montorsi F, Mulhall JP, Stief C. Prevention and management of post-prostatectomy sexual dysfunctions part 2: recovery and preservation of erectile function, sexual desire, and orgasmic function. Eur Urol. 2012;62(2):273–86.
25. Ronchetti C, Cirillo F, Di Segni N, et al. Inflammatory bowel disease and reproductive health: from fertility to pregnancy: a narrative review. Nutrients. 2022;14:1591. https://doi.org/10.3390/nu14081591.
26. Bertani L, Ribaldone DG, Bellini M, et al. Inflammatory bowel diseases: is there a role for nutritional suggestions? Nutrients. 2021;13:1387. https://doi.org/10.3390/nu13041387.
27. Ananthakrishnan AN, Kaplan GG, Bernstein CN, et al. Lifestyle, behavior, and environmental modification for management of patients with inflammatory bowel disease: a consensus from the International Organization for the Study of inflammatory bowel diseases. Lancet Gastroenterol Hepatol. 2022;7:666–78. https://doi.org/10.1016/S2468-1253(22)00021-8.
28. Mantzouranis G, Fafliora E, Glanztounis G, et al. Inflammatory bowel disease and sexual function in male and female patients: an update on evidence in the last ten years. J Crohns Colitis. 2015;9:1160–8. https://doi.org/10.1093/ecco-jcc/jjv140.
29. Knowles SR, Gass C, Macrae F. Disease perception in IBD influences psychological status, sexual health and satisfaction, body image, and relational functioning: a preliminary exploration using structural equation modeling. J Crohns Colitis. 2013;7:e344–50. https://doi.org/10.1016/j.crohns.2013.01.018.

30. Mahmood S, Nusrat S, Crosby A, et al. Evaluation of sexual function among patients with inflammatory bowel disease. Am J Gastroenterol. 2015;110:601–3. https://doi.org/10.1038/ajg.2015.53.
31. Eluri S, Cross RK, Martin C, et al. Inflammatory bowel diseases can negatively impact domains of sexual function, such as satisfaction with sex life. Dig Dis Sci. 2018;63:1572–82. https://doi.org/10.1007/s10620-018-5021-8.
32. Chen B, Zhou B, Song G, Li H, Li R, Liu Z, Wei C, Wang T, Wang S, Ma D, Liu J, Yuan X, Liu X. Inflammatory bowel disease is associated with worse sexual function: a systematic review and meta-analysis. Transl Androl Urol. 2022;11(7):959–73.
33. Perez de Arce E, Quera R, Ribeiro Barros J, et al. Sexual dysfunction in inflammatory bowel disease: what the specialist should know and ask. Int J Gen Med. 2021;14:2003–15. https://doi.org/10.2147/IJGM.S308214.
34. Shmidt E, Suárez-Fariñas M, Mallette M, et al. Erectile dysfunction is highly prevalent in men with newly diagnosed inflammatory bowel disease. Inflamm Bowel Dis. 2019;25(8):1408–16.
35. Timmer A, Bauer A, Kemptner D, Furst A, Rogler G. Determinants of male sexual function in inflammatory bowel disease: a cross-sectional analysis based on a survey in 280 men. Inflamm Bowel Dis. 2007;13(10):1236–43. https://doi.org/10.1002/ibd.20182.
36. Marín L, Mañosa M, Garcia-Planella E, et al. Sexual function and patient perceptions in inflammatory bowel disease: a case-control survey. J Gastroenterol. 2013;48(6):713–20. https://doi.org/10.1007/s00535-012-0700-2.
37. Muller KR, Prosser R, Bampton P, Mountifield R, Andrews JM. Female gender and surgery compromise relationships, body image and sexuality in inflammatory bowel disease: patient perceptions. Inflamm Bowel Dis. 2010;16(4):657–63. https://doi.org/10.1002/ibd.21090.
38. Grimstad T, Norheim KB, Isaksen K, et al. Fatigue in newly diagnosed inflammatory bowel disease. J Crohns Colitis. 2015;9(9):725–30. https://doi.org/10.1093/ecco-jcc/jjv091.
39. Nocerino A, Nguyen A, Agrawal M, Mone A, Lakhani K, Swaminath A. Fatigue in inflammatory bowel diseases: etiologies and management. Adv Ther. 2020;37(1):97–112. https://doi.org/10.1007/s12325-019-01151-w.
40. Romberg-Camps MJ, Bol Y, Dagnelie PC. Fatigue and health-related quality of life in inflammatory bowel disease: results from a population-based study in The Netherlands: the IBD-South Limburg cohort. Inflamm Bowel Dis. 2010;16(12):2137–47. https://doi.org/10.1002/ibd.21285.
41. Maunder R, Toner B, de Rooy E, Moskovitz D. Influence of sex and disease on illness-related concerns in inflammatory bowel disease. Can J Gastroenterol. 1999;13(9):728–32. https://doi.org/10.1155/1999/701645.
42. Malavige LS, Jayaratne SD, Kathriarachchi ST, Sivayogan S, Fernando DJ, Levy JC. Erectile dysfunction among men with diabetes is strongly associated with premature ejaculation and reduced libido. J Sex Med. 2008;5:2125–34.
43. Yu LW, Kong AP, Tong PC, Tam C, Ko GT, Ho CS, et al. Evaluation of erectile dysfunction and associated cardiovascular risk using structured questionnaires in Chinese men with type 2 diabetes. Int J Androl. 2010;33:853–60.

Part II

Clinical and Therapeutic Approaches

Clinical and Pharmacological Approaches to Hypoactive Sexual Desire Disorder in Humans

5

Abstract

The scientific discussion is ongoing regarding whether desire and arousal can be reliably differentiated in men, and parallels are drawn with the literature on women. Generally, three options are hypothesized for the diagnosis of low desire in men for the DSM-5. **Option 1** proposes that the name and criteria of DSM-IV-TR be retained for men in DSM-5. **Option 2** suggests adopting the recently proposed criteria for the disorder of sexual interest and arousal in women for men, which would result in a gender-neutral category. **Option 3** recommends applying the criteria for the disorder of sexual interest and arousal to men, with a small modification to one criterion: namely, that the absent or reduced genital and non-genital physical changes are not included as a criterion. This diagnosis would only be applied to men (Brotto LA. J Sex Med 7:2015–2030, 2010).

Keywords

Hypoactive sexual desire disorder · Sexual interest · Sexual desire · DSM diagnostic criteria · Kinase inhibitors · Receptor modulators · Buchwald-Hartwig amination · Aromatic nucleophilic substitution · Reductive amination · Finkelstein alkylation · Amide bond formation · Self-administered questionnaires

5.1 Introduction

Pharmacological research has identified in **flibanserin** unique properties and selective agonist and antagonist activity against serotonin receptors. Originally, its primary application was in the treatment of hypoactive sexual desire disorder (HSDD) in women, where it showed promising results in improving sexual desire. However, with the expansion of understanding of its mechanism of action, researchers have begun to explore its potential usefulness in the treatment of HSDD in men.

E. V. Longhi, *Hypoactive Sexual Desire Disorder*,
https://doi.org/10.1007/978-3-032-00659-2_5

This emerging trend has led to a growing interest in the use of *flibanserin* as a potential therapeutic option for men experiencing a decrease in sexual desire.

A retrospective analysis was conducted G Saffati et al., [1] which included a cohort of men who had started treatment with flibanserin **between July 2022 and July 2023**. Basic demographic information was collected, including total and free testosterone levels, relevant medical history, scores of the *International Index of Erectile Function* (IIEF), the *Patient Health Questionnaire-9* (PHQ-9), and overall manifestation of side effects.

A total of 26 patients were identified, with an average age of 57.9 years (range, 31–80 years). Among these patients, seven had a previous diagnosis of depression and had previously received treatment with selective serotonin reuptake inhibitors (SSRIs). The average levels of total testosterone and free testosterone were found to be 611.3 ng/dL and 116.8 pg/mL, respectively. Notably, a significant majority of patients (22 out of 26, 81.4%) were diagnosed with erectile dysfunction.

It is important to note that all patients presented in a euthyroid state.

The average baseline score on the PHQ-9 was 5.30 (range, 0–17), indicating mild depressive symptoms, while the average total IIEF score was 40 (range, 6–67). *Moreover, the average score on the IIEF-desire subdomain was 5.65, reflecting relatively reduced levels of sexual desire.*

After conducting a follow-up evaluation at the third month, it was observed that seven patients discontinued flibanserin therapy, with reasons such as inefficacy and high costs cited as primary factors. Notably, only one patient (3.8%) discontinued therapy due to side effects.

This research has clarified the fundamental characteristics associated with off-label use of flibanserin in men with HSDD, highlighting the growing interest in investigating its potential therapeutic benefits within this specific population. However, further research is needed to comprehensively clarify the clinical benefits and potential risks of administering flibanserin in men.

5.2 Safety Evaluation of "Flibanserin"

Although approved by the U.S. Food and Drug Administration (FDA) for the treatment of generalized hypoactive sexual desire disorder, there are doubts and perplexities. *During the FDA review of flibanserin, concerns were raised regarding the risks of hypotension, syncope, and adverse events related to sedation, which increase with alcohol use.* Based on the results of an alcohol provocation study, the FDA has required a boxed warning and a contraindication to alcohol in the prescribing information for flibanserin, as part of a risk evaluation and mitigation strategy program [2].

This was a review of the data provided in the product prescribing information for flibanserin, selective serotonin reuptake inhibitors, serotonin-norepinephrine reuptake inhibitors, other serotonergic antidepressants, and triptans.

The incidences of hypotension, syncope, and adverse events related to sedation (for example, dizziness, drowsiness, fatigue) in flibanserin studies fell within the ranges observed for serotonergic antidepressants; the rates of these adverse events were generally lower with triptan drugs. Other adverse events associated with flibanserin (for example, nausea, insomnia, dry mouth) occurred more commonly in patients taking antidepressant drugs.

Although drugs that affect the serotonin system present variable adverse event profiles (likely mediated by differences in serotonin-related mechanisms of action, specific brain structures involved, and effects on other neurotransmitter systems), the occurrence of central nervous system-related adverse events was not dissimilar between flibanserin and serotonergic antidepressants.

A post hoc analysis of the data from HSDD clinical studies found that treatment with flibanserin was associated with a statistically significant weight loss compared to placebo, even though the study patients were not selected to be overweight or obese and had not received any expectation of weight reduction or interventions aimed at promoting weight loss.

A literature review was conducted using the *Medline* database for relevant publications on the mechanisms of action through which flibanserin may promote weight loss and on the links between sexual function and weight management [3].

Based on the data from the clinical studies on flibanserin, there was no consistent correlation between weight loss and improvement in sexual function, as assessed by HSDD outcome measures. Even nausea, a common adverse event associated with the use of flibanserin, did not appear to be a factor contributing to weight loss. Hypothetical links between flibanserin treatment and weight loss include modulation of peripheral 5-HT2A receptors and factors such as improved mood and sleep.

The study by Clayton AH et al. [4] investigated the pharmacokinetics of *flibanserin*, the proposed mechanism of action, and safety data in clinical studies with a focus on sedation and hypotension-related adverse events, as well as pharmacological interactions with alcohol and antidepressants. The sources included peer-reviewed publications and internal manufacturer data.

Before flibanserin, there were no approved drugs for the treatment of hypoactive sexual desire disorder. To study the efficacy of flibanserin, the FDA required satisfying sexual events as the primary endpoint, although this endpoint does not measure the level of desire or associated discomfort. The measurement of the satisfying sexual events was significant in all three flibanserin studies.

Safety concerns focused on the incidence of sedation, syncope, hypotension, and the interaction of flibanserin with alcohol and CYP3A4 inhibitors. Further targeted provocation studies were required by the FDA [5].

The *Food and Drug Administration* (FDA) in the United States has approved two drugs for "hypoactive sexual desire disorder" flibanserin (Addyi) in 2015 and **bremelanotide** (Vyleesi) in 2019. In clinical studies, flibanserin led to an average of only one additional enjoyable sexual experience every 2 months; bremelanotide to none. The studies for both drugs present changes in primary outcomes and a contested indication. A politicized, industry-sponsored advocacy campaign and contrasting testimonies from patients and experts likely influenced the approval of flibanserin on its third attempt. Bremelanotide, with even weaker efficacy, capitalized on the regulatory precedent set by the approval of flibanserin [6].

The study by Cipriani S. et al. [7] examined the proposed mechanism of action of *bremelanotide*, the pharmacokinetics, efficacy, and safety data derived from clinical studies. A literature search of peer-reviewed publications on the current evidence regarding bremelanotide pharmacotherapy was performed using the *PubMed* database.

Bremelanotide appears to be moderately safe and well tolerated; the most common adverse reaction is nausea (40%). Although the data from clinical studies have shown a significant change in the validated questionnaires, the overall clinical benefit appears to be modest. However, these results should be interpreted in light of the dramatic challenges in conducting well-designed clinical studies for HSDD, due to the significant placebo effect of pharmacotherapy and the frequent use of outcome measures that are likely highly susceptible to expectation bias—such as long recall periods for sexual and emotional response.

The efficacy and safety of bremelanotide, a melanocortin receptor agonist approved by the U.S. Food and Drug Administration for the treatment of generalized HSDD, have been established in the Phase 3 *RECONNECT* studies, two randomized, double-blind, placebo-controlled studies designed identically with an optional 52-week open-label extension. This report examines the efficacy of bremelanotide versus placebo based on predefined subgroups [age, weight, body mass index (BMI), and bioavailable testosterone] in the RECONNECT studies [8].

Patients self-administered bremelanotide 1.75 mg or placebo subcutaneously, using an autoinjector, as needed, before sexual activity for 24 weeks. Efficacy was assessed based on the change from baseline to the end of the study for the desire domain of the *Female Sexual Function Index* and the *Female Sexual Distress Scale—Desire/Arousal/Orgasm* item 13 for *bremelanotide* versus placebo.

Among the **1754** patients included in the integrated and subgroup analyses, *bremelanotide* achieved statistically significant improvements in measures of increased desire and decreased distress associated with low desire in all age, weight, and BMI subgroups and all quartiles of baseline bioavailable testosterone, with few exceptions.

Bremelanotide was further associated with statistically significant increases in reported sexual desire in patients not taking hormonal contraceptives, and with a numerical advantage in those taking hormonal contraceptives. Statistically significant improvements were observed regardless of the presence or absence of reduced arousal and the duration of HSDD. According to some scientific hypotheses, these female evaluations of bremelanotide could also be applied to men affected by HSDD.

That said, despite the high prevalence of low sexual desire, knowledge about its predictive factors and their importance in onset is limited. The purpose of the study by Rastrelli G. et al. [9] was to identify the factors that predispose to reduced sexual desire or hypoactive sexual desire (HSD) characterized by patient distress (HSDD). This is a prospective observational cohort study with a median follow-up of 4.3 years.

A total of 3369 men aged between 40 and 79 were recruited through eight European clinical research centers. Among the studied subjects, 456 (20.1%) reported having developed or worsened the level of their sexual desire during the follow-up period, while 214 (9.5%) reported new-onset or worsening HSDD. Potential predictors, categorized into three clusters (objective parameters; subjective parameters; sexual symptoms and relational conditions), were analyzed and evaluated through multiple regression models.

Low sexual desire and HSDD, while sharing some predictors, shows important differences. A low level of total or free testosterone predicted the decline of the frequency of sexual thoughts (OR = 1.7[1.2–2.4] and 1.5[1.1–2.0], respectively). Other predictors of the decline of sexual thoughts included the presence of comorbidities, lower cognitive function, and physical inactivity. Conversely, HSDD was not predicted by androgens; its main predictors were visceral obesity.

5.3 Psychosexual Treatments

Publications support the efficacy of the treatment of hypoactive sexual desire disorder (HSDD) in women and men with cognitive-behavioral therapy (CBT) and mindfulness meditation training (MMT). However, no review has evaluated the scientific evidence for these therapies from the rigorous perspective of sexual medicine.

The study by Robert E. Pyke et al. [10] evaluated the published controlled clinical studies on cognitive-behavioral therapy and mindfulness meditation training for sexual desire disorders from the standpoint of sexual medicine control standards, risk/benefit ratios, and clinical significance.

Studies were evaluated through *MEDLINE* over the past 10 years. The quality of the studies was assessed using 10 parameters, and efficacy was measured as the average change, as well as the proportion of responders and remitters.

Three controlled studies support cognitive-behavioral therapy (CBT), and two controlled studies support MMT. However, the study reports lacked several scientific requirements: a hierarchy of endpoints with a planned primary endpoint, sufficient information on the intervention to reproduce it, randomization, adequate control, accepted measures of benefits and harms, compliance data, and/or results of clinical relevance.

However, the study by Cipriani, S., et al. [11] evaluated the relationship between female sexual dysfunction (FSD) and eating disorders (ED). This hypothesis can be compared with other studies on hypoactive sexual desire disorder (HSDD) and male sexual dysfunctions. One hundred and twenty-three women retrospectively recruited for a consultation on FSD underwent a medical examination and completed the following validated questionnaires: *Female Sexual Function Index* (FSFI), *Female Sexual Distress Scale-Revised* (FSDS-R), *Eating Disorder Examination Questionnaire* (EDE-Q), *Binge Eating Scale* (BES), *Emotional Eating Scale* (EES), *Barrat Impulsiveness Scale-11* (BIS-11), *Beck Depression Inventory* (BDI), *State-Trait Anxiety Inventory Y* (STAI Y), *Symptom Checklist 90-Revised* (SCL-90-R), *Body Uneasiness Test* (BUT), *Dyadic Adjustment Scale* (DAS), and *Sexual Inhibition/Sexual Excitation Scales (SIS/SES)*.

Additionally, demographic, medical, and psychosexual data were obtained through a structured interview.

When patients were classified by BMI (<25, 25–30, >30 kg/m2), it emerged that all scores related to the EDE-Q subscales were significantly different among the three subgroups (all $p \leq 0.001$).

Furthermore, patients with a history of unwanted sexual experiences (USE) had significantly higher total BES ($p = 0.034$) and EES ($p = 0.027$) scores compared to those without. Also, when examining patients based on the clinical diagnosis of hypoactive sexual desire disorder (HSDD), it emerged that individuals with HSDD showed a worse psychological profile compared to those without, particularly a higher score on EDE-Q and BDI (all $p \leq 0.05$). Moreover, when examining patients for the other two main diagnoses of FSD, female genital arousal disorder (FGAD) and female orgasm disorder (FOD), no significant differences were observed among all the examined questionnaires.

To further verify the impact of different psychopathological aspects on the risk of having HSDD, it emerged that the only questionnaire scores that contributed to this dysfunction were EDE-Q, total BDI, and SIS1 after age adjustment. Finally, patients were evaluated in three groups: no binge eating (BE), sporadic BE, and frequent BE, observing a significant positive association between BE frequency and sexual distress, as evaluated by the total FSDS-R score.

In conclusion, in a population of women affected by FSD, ED traits could negatively influence sexual desire, representing a significant risk factor for the clinical diagnosis of HSDD. Among all the psychopathological aspects investigated, psychological alterations related to ED seem to have a more pronounced effect on HSDD compared to other commonly accepted risk factors for sexual desire disorders, such as depression and increased inhibitory trait. From a clinical perspective, it would be worth investigating these findings also in andrological settings.

5.3.1 Metacognitive Therapy

A new clinical psychotherapy study for patients with *Hypoactive Sexual Desire Disorder* (HSDD), according to the *Diagnostic and Statistical Manual of Mental Disorders*, fourth edition, has recently been published. Significant benefits with metacognitive therapy (MCT), a widely tested process for treating depression and anxiety that had not previously been tested for psychosexual disorders, were highlighted [12].

Metacognition is thinking about thinking—observing one's thoughts and monitoring, controlling, and evaluating them. Apparently, MCT works for depression and anxiety by showing patients how their repetitive negative thoughts, worries, and ruminations are counterproductive; thus, patients are taught to use metacognitive strategies to replace their beliefs and negative ways of thinking. In practice, the patient is encouraged to build only on neutral or positive thoughts. This approach seems similar to a multifaceted psychotherapeutic method that has been specifically adapted to treat HSDD: mindfulness-based reflection training integrated with cognitive-behavioral therapy. However, the logic hypothesized is that such a general and personally non-invasive approach could be useful for managing overarching thought processes rather than delving into explicit sexual content or behaviors. Furthermore, the generality of this approach could have facilitated acceptance. The researchers in question were treating patients in Iran.

5.4 Operational Procedures for HSDD in Men

The study by Eusebio Rubio-Aurioles et al. [13] attempted to outline diagnostic guidelines for hypoactive sexual desire disorder in men.

A review of the scientific literature reveals a new classification scheme; LSD/I is proposed as a generic term for which hypoactive sexual desire disorder (HSDD) is just a subtype. The following standard operating procedures are described: *(i) detection of LSD/I: screening for LSD/I, screening for LSD/I in patients with other sexual dysfunctions; (ii) diagnosis and assessment of etiology: diagnostic criteria for LSD/I, assessment of depression status, assessment of relationship status, assessment of endocrine status, diagnostic criteria for HSDD in men; (iii) treatment: treatment of LSD/I secondary to low testosterone, treatment of LSD/I secondary to elevated prolactin, treatment of LSD/I secondary to other endocrine disorders, treatment of LSD/I secondary to depressive illness and/or anxiety disorders, treatment of LSD/I secondary to relational conflict, and treatment of HSDD. A diagnostic and treatment algorithm is presented.*

Once the diagnosis of LSD/I in men is confirmed, a thorough search for possible causes should include both biological and psychological factors. The treatment should be etiologically oriented.

According to the model of interpersonal emotion regulation of sexual dysfunction, the way couples manage their emotions in relation to sexual problems can promote or hinder sexual communication. In the first dyadic study to date on men with HSDD and their partners (64 couples), the associations between two emotion regulation strategies—*reappraisal and suppression*—and the *couples' communication about their sexual relationship* were studied. Participants completed measures assessing the use of reappraisal and suppression in their sexual relationship, sexual communication, and sexual assertiveness. Men with HSDD who reported greater suppression also reported *lower sexual assertiveness*, and both partners reported poorer sexual communication. The partners of men with HSDD who used greater suppression were less sexually assertive. Conversely, while reappraisal was only marginally associated with the perceived quality of sexual communication, men with *HSDD* who employed more reappraisal were also more sexually assertive. Although suppression may hinder sexual communication, reappraisal may enable men with HSDD to better assert their sexual needs. The results can inform interventions to help couples manage impactful emotional experiences associated with HSDD [14].

For the completeness of the study by McClung E et al. [15], it was shown that, despite their low desire, *men with HSDD often reported desiring sexual intimacy and validation within their sexual relationships*. Studies applying self-determination theory to sexual relationships show that adopting more autonomous motivations—engaging in sex for its intrinsic pleasure—and less self-competitive motivations—experiencing sexuality for a reward or partner satisfaction—result in greater sexual well-being for both members of the couple.

Since autonomous motivation in relationships is associated with intimacy, sexual satisfaction, and less sexual discomfort, experiencing a sexual relationship *for autonomous reasons may allow men with HSDD and their partners to feel more sexually intimate despite their lower sexual desire*.

In this cross-sectional dyadic study [15], the associations between *types of sexual motivation and sexual intimacy, sexual satisfaction, and sexual discomfort for men with HSDD and their partners—64 couples*—were studied.

Men with HSDD who reported experiencing intimacy for more autonomous reasons reported greater sexual satisfaction, and both partners reported greater sexual intimacy.

Men with HSDD who experienced sexuality for more controlled reasons had partners who experienced less intimacy and sexual satisfaction, and both partners were more sexually stressed.

The fact remains that the psychosexual approach shows more adaptive results for the patient and the partner.

HSDD is present in 8.9% of women aged 18–44, in 12.3% aged 45–64, and in 7.4% over 65 years of age. Although low sexual desire increases with age, discomfort decreases; therefore, the prevalence of HSDD remains relatively constant based on age. HSDD is associated with lower health-related quality of life, less happiness and overall satisfaction with partners, and more frequent negative emotional states. **HSDD is underdiagnosed and undertreated**. Less than half of patients with sexual problems seek help or initiate discussions with doctors. *Patients are inhibited by the fear of embarrassing doctors and believe that doctors should initiate the discussions*. The *Decreased Sexual Desire Screener*, a tool for detecting and diagnosing HSDD, is validated for use in general medicine.

But the sexologist goes further. To make communication more fluid, we must always remember that the doctor-patient relationship depends on three variables: context, patient, and doctor.

The relationship is influenced by the place where it is experienced, by the psychological structure of the patient, by the pathology they suffer from, by the anxiety inherent in a surgical intervention, by the doctor's attitude towards welcoming individuals, and by the goal set by the specialist.

The first visit or the first medical patient approach shows different characteristics depending on whether it takes place in a *university health facility* or in *private practice*.

As I described in one of my publications [16], immediately addressing the pathology in a quick and concise manner could cause dissatisfaction in the patient and doubts about the diagnosis and the proposed surgical path.

In a private context, the patient assumes they will be welcomed into a hospitable, depathologizing, non-anxiety-inducing environment with a secretarial team that offers empathy, availability and kindness.

Human contact is more immediate and less forced during a first visit, during which the patient, usually feels more free to express their concerns, symptoms, and emotions—without the anxiety of the limited time allowed for a typical visit to a university facility.

In any case, it is essential to observe the patient's attitude toward the "disease': what idea have they formed of HSDD? Do they exaggerate, dramatize, or minimize? And what about the partner?

Nine areas of psychosexual investigation:

(a) Personality and sensitivity of the patient.
(b) Codification of relationships (previous partner, family of origin, friends, etc.) that they have best understood.
(c) Body map awareness.
(d) Quality of life of the individual.
(e) Quality of life of the couple.
(f) Quality of life in the family of origin.
(g) View of the future.
(h) Expectations of the doctor-patient relationship.
(i) Expectations of the sexologist-patient relationship.

One study from the UK found that among 6777 sexually active women, 34.2% experienced low desire [17]. Applying the morbidity criteria listed in the fifth edition of the *Diagnostic and Statistical Manual of Mental Disorders* (DSM-5), 6.5% of women indicated low desire or sexual arousal for several months in the past year, and 0.6% met the criteria for female sexual interest/arousal disorder [18]. Low sexual desire not only affects women's sexual health, but also has negative effects on their quality of life [19]. Individuals with sexual dysfunctions—including low desire—are more likely to report higher rates of sexually transmitted infections, unwanted sex, unemployment, relationship breakdown, and difficulty discussing sexuality. Moreover, low sexual desire is often linked to mental health problems such as depression and anxiety.

Although many individuals—both men and women—are distressed by the lack of desire, the number of those receiving qualified, evidence-based treatment remains low [20]. Sexual dysfunctions are linked to stigma and reluctance to seek professional help [21]. Moreover, there is a prevailing lack of information on treatment options and structural barriers, such as limited access to qualified therapists. This problem could be addressed by developing and disseminating treatments that require less direct contact, namely Internet-Based interventions. A growing body of literature suggests that interventions provided via the Internet or mobile technology are feasible and effective for improving depression, anxiety, and even psychosis [22]. These interventions offer various degrees of guidance, ranging from self-help to user-guided interventions to regular contact with a qualified clinician. Interventions involving at least some guidance or coaching have proven to be more effective than unguided interventions [23]. Regarding Internet-Based interventions for sexual dysfunctions in women, van Lankveld et al. [24] examined five studies and found that these interventions were effective in improving sexual functioning and emotional intimacy in couples. While two of these studies also included women with low sexual desire, the treatments did not focus solely on improving sexual desire but targeted a wide range of women's sexual difficulties—for example, anorgasmia and genital pain. Therefore, no study has evaluated the effectiveness of *Cognitive Behavioral Therapy* (CBT) based on Internet (I-CBT) or mindfulness-based therapy (I-MBT) designed specifically for the treatment of low sexual desire in women.

5.5 Conclusions

A systematic review was conducted in the *PubMed*, *EMBASE*, *PsycINFO*, *Science Direct*, and *Web of Science* databases [25]. The search yielded 1203 articles, of which 15 were included in the review. It identified ten tools originally developed in English.

Regarding desire and sexual functioning, several questionnaires applied to the diagnosis of hypoactive sexual desire disorder and estimating their actual prevalence, associated factors, and their extent were observed [26]. Out of a total of 1203 identified articles, 21 were included in the review, in which ten tools were identified.

Also, the aim of the *COnsensus-based Standards for the selection of health status Measurement INstruments* (COSMIN) study was to develop a consensus-based checklist to assess the methodological quality of studies on measurement properties.

In this case, a four-round Delphi study was conducted with international experts—psychologists, epidemiologists, statisticians, and clinicians. Of the 91 experts invited, 57 agreed to participate (63%). Panel members were asked to rate their "(dis)agreement" with each proposal on a five-point scale. Consensus was considered reached when at least 67% of panel members indicated "agree" or "strongly agree" [27].

Consensus was reached on the inclusion of the following measurement properties: *internal consistency, reliability, measurement error, content validity (including face validity), construct validity (including structural validity, hypothesis testing, and cross-cultural validity), criterion validity, responsiveness, and interpretability*. The panel also reached consensus on how these properties should be evaluated.

The resulting *COSMIN* checklist could be useful in choosing a measurement tool, in peer review of a manuscript, in designing or communicating a study on measurement properties, or for educational purposes.

In conclusion, scientific studies delve into the possibility of thoroughly understanding hypoactive sexual desire disorder, especially in male patients.

In the therapeutic field, however, it should be emphasized that, in addition to scientific professionalism, it is necessary to enhance the communicative empathy of doctors and psychosocial accompaniment alongside pharmacology.

The andrologist-psychologist team does not induce perplexity or mistrust in the patient and partner. Rather, the excessive use of medical terms in communication and the disproportionate use of diagnostic tools pathologize not only the patient but also compromise the therapeutic process. The individual and the couple need synergistic clinical-sexological accompaniment for effective care and better compliance in the therapeutic process. Seventy percent of therapeutic success depends on the communicative style of the doctor-patient-sexologist.

References

1. Saffati G, Naeem T, La TM, Kaaki B, Khera M. (166) Safety of flibanserin in men with hypoactive sexual desire disorder. J Sex Med. 2024;21(Supplement_1)., qdae001.157. https://doi.org/10.1093/jsxmed/qdae001.157.
2. Kingsberg SA, McElroy SL, Clayton AH. Evaluation of Flibanserin safety: comparison with other serotonergic medications. Sex Med Rev. 2019;7(3):380–92.
3. Simon JA, Kingsberg SA, Goldstein I, Kim NN, Hakim B, Millheiser L. Weight loss in women taking Flibanserin for hypoactive sexual desire disorder (HSDD): insights into potential mechanisms. Sex Med Rev. 2019;7(4):575–86.
4. Clayton AH, Brown L, Kim NN. Evaluation of safety for flibanserin. Expert Opin Drug Saf. 2020;19(1):1–8.
5. Dooley EM, Miller MK, Clayton AH. Flibanserin: from bench to bedside. Sex Med Rev. 2017;5(4):461–9. https://doi.org/10.1016/j.sxmr.2017.06.003. Epub 2017 Jul 27. PMID: 28757356.
6. Mintzes B, Tiefer L, Cosgrove L. Bremelanotide and flibanserin for low sexual desire in women: the fallacy of regulatory precedent. Drug Ther Bull. 2021;59(12):185–8.
7. Cipriani S, Alfaroli C, Maseroli E, Vignozzi L. An evaluation of bremelanotide injection for the treatment of hypoactive sexual desire disorder. Expert Opin Pharmacother. 2023;24(1):15–21.
8. Simon JA, Kingsberg SA, Portman D, Jordan R, Lucas J, Sadiq A, Krop J, Clayton AH. Prespecified and integrated subgroup analyses from the RECONNECT Phase 3 studies of Bremelanotide. J Womens Health (Larchmt). 2022;31(3):391–400.
9. Rastrelli G, O'Neill T, Corona G, Bartfai G, Casanueva F, Forti G, Vanderschueren D, Slowikowska-Hilczer J, Giwercman A, Punab M, Huhtaniemi I, Wu F, Maggi M. EMAS group, PS-8-6 predictors of sexual desire decline or development of hypoactive sexual desire disorder: longitudinal results from the European male aging study. J Sex Med. 2020;17(Supplement_2):S145. https://doi.org/10.1016/j.jsxm.2020.04.080.
10. Pyke RE, Clayton AH. Trials of psychological treatment for hypoactive sexual desire disorder: a critique and a perspective from sexual medicine. J Sex Med. 2015;12(12):2451–8. https://doi.org/10.1111/jsm.13056.
11. Cipriani S, Maseroli E, Di Stasi V, Scavello I, Paoletti C, Castellini G, Ricca V, Maggi M, Vignozzi L. 107 eating disorder symptoms as a risk factor for hypoactive sexual desire disorder in women: a pilot-study. J Sex Med. 2022;19(Supplement_2):S167. https://doi.org/10.1016/j.jsxm.2022.03.381.
12. Pyke RE. Metacognitive therapy trial for hypoactive sexual desire disorder breaks the Mold. J Sex Med. 2017;14(12):1629–30. https://doi.org/10.1016/j.jsxm.2017.10.069.
13. Rubio-Aurioles E, Bivalacqua TJ. Standard operative procedures for low sexual desire in men. J Sex Med. 2013;10(1):94–107. https://doi.org/10.1111/j.1743-6109.2012.02778.x.
14. Wang GA, Corsini-Munt S, Dubé JP, McClung E, Rosen NO. Regulate and communicate: associations between emotion regulation and sexual communication among men with hypoactive sexual desire disorder and their partners. J Sex Res. 2023;60(3):325–35.
15. McClung E, Rosen NO, Dubé JP, Wang GA, Corsini-Munt S. Motivation when desire is low: associations between sexual motivation and sexual intimacy, sexual satisfaction, and sexual distress for men with hypoactive sexual desire disorder and their partners. Arch Sex Behav. 2024;53(3):1075–89.
16. Longhi EV, Franco G, Colombo F. Psychosexual counseling in andrological surgery. Springer; 2000.

17. Mitchell KR, Mercer CH, Ploubidis GB, Jones KG, Datta J, Field N, Copas AJ, Tanton C, Erens B, Sonnenberg P, Clifton S, Macdowall W, Phelps A, Johnson AM, Wellings K. Sexual function in Great Britain: findings from the third National Survey of Sexual Attitudes and Lifestyles (Natsal-3). Lancet. 2013;382(9907):1817–29.
18. Mitchell KR, Jones KG, Wellings K, Johnson AM, Graham CA, Datta J, Copas AJ, Bancroft J, Sonnenberg P, Macdowall W, Field N, Mercer CH. Estimating the prevalence of sexual function problems: the impact of morbidity criteria. J Sex Res. 2016;53(8):955–67.
19. Biddle AK, West SL, D'Aloisio AA, Wheeler SB, Borisov NN, Thorp J. Hypoactive sexual desire disorder in postmenopausal women: quality of life and health impact. Value Health. 2009;12(5):763–72.
20. Parish SJ, Hahn SR. Hypoactive sexual desire disorder: a review of epidemiology, biopsychology, diagnosis, and treatment. Sex Med Rev. 2016;4(2):103–20.
21. Velten J, Pantazidis P, Benecke A, Fehm AK, Bräscher L, Fladung AK, Fydrich T, Heider J, Hamm A, InAlbon T, Lange J, Lincoln T, Lutz W, Margraf J, Schlarb A, Schöttke H, Trösken A, Weinmann-Lutz B, Hoyer J. How often are diagnoses in the field of sexual dysfunction assigned at German university outpatient clinics for psychotherapy at psychological institutes? J Sex, Research. 2020;
22. Alvarez-Jimenez M, Alcazar-Corcoles MA, González-Blanch C, Bendall S, McGorry PD, Gleeson JF. Online technologies, social media, and mobile for the treatment of psychosis: a systematic review on new user-guided interventions. Schizophr Res. 2014;156(1):96–106.
23. Berger T. The therapeutic alliance in internet interventions: a narrative review and suggestions for future research. Psychother Res. 2017;27(5):511–24.
24. van Lankveld J. Internet-based interventions for female sexual dysfunction. Curr Sex Health Rep. 2016;8:136–43. https://doi.org/10.1007/s11930-016-0087-9. http://europepmc.org/abstract/MED/27512346.
25. Cartagena-Ramos D, Fuentealba-Torres M, Rebustini F, Leite ACAB, Alvarenga WA, Arcêncio RA, Dantas RAS, Nascimento LC. Systematic review of the psychometric properties of instruments to measure sexual desire. BMC Med Res Methodol. 2018;18(1):109.
26. McCool ME, Zuelke A, Theurich MA, Knuettel H, Ricci C, Apfelbacher C. Prevalence of female sexual dysfunction among premenopausal women: a systematic review and meta-analysis of observational studies. Sex Med Rev. 2016;4:197–212.
27. Mokkink LB, Terwee CB, Patrick DL, Alonso J, Stratford PW, Knol DL, Bouter LM, de Vet HC. The COSMIN checklist for assessing the methodological quality of studies on measurement properties of health status measurement instruments: an international Delphi study. Qual Life Res. 2010;19(4):539–49.

Impact of Hypoactive Sexual Desire Disorders on Mental Well-Being and Daily Activities: Pharmacological Therapy?

6

Abstract

It has been found that the symptomatic burden of HSDD is negatively and statistically significantly associated with patients' mental health; the impact was greater among premenopausal women compared to those in postmenopause. However, although HSDD affects the quality of life and interpersonal relationships of the patient, **the disorder often goes unaddressed or untreated**. Recent studies on the disease burden in women with HSDD, particularly in premenopausal women, are limited.

Keywords

Female sexual dysfunction · Hypoactive sexual desire disorder · Mental health · Quality of life · Premenopause · Body weight · Flibanserin · Reproductive health · Sexuality · Weight loss · Bremelanotide

6.1 Introduction

A cross-sectional study [1] has shown that *about one in ten women in the United States suffers from low sexual desire and associated distress: HSDD affects 8.9% of women aged between 18 and 44 years, 12.3% of women aged between 45 and 65 years, and 7.4% of women aged 65 years or older*. Although HSDD impacts women's health-related quality of life (HRQoL), the disorder often goes unaddressed or untreated [2].

Women may delay or not seek treatment for HSDD for various reasons, including the belief that their sexual difficulties are temporary and will resolve; that their experience is a normal part of aging or long-term relationships; an aversion to discussing what they see as a private or embarrassing issue; and uncertainty about where to seek help [3]. Moreover, physicians who frequently treat HSDD, such as general practitioners and obstetricians-gynecologists, often show hesitation in

E. V. Longhi, *Hypoactive Sexual Desire Disorder*,
https://doi.org/10.1007/978-3-032-00659-2_6

addressing sexual health due to concerns about causing discomfort in their relationships with patients and the underlying attitudes of the physicians themselves towards sexuality [4].

In this regard, the study conducted by Simon JA et al. [5] recruited on the web **32,178** participants online 1508 (4.6%) were diagnosed with HSDD, 1108 (3.4%) were diagnosed with HSDD by a physician; and 418 (1.3%) qualified based on DSDS criteria.

Of these 1508 participants, 857 (50%) met the eligibility requirements to participate in the study, and 530 (62%) completed the survey and were included in the study analyses.

Most participants were premenopausal, married, Caucasian, college-educated, and in a heterosexual relationship.

Among all participants, 75% reported having spoken with a physician or therapist about HSDD symptoms, while 25% did not. Among those who spoke with a physician or therapist, 82% initiated the conversation with their healthcare provider (HCP). On average, it took 10 months for participants to see a physician after experiencing the initial symptoms of HSDD, with a delay of about 2 months in the diagnosis of HSDD.

6.2 Reluctance to Report HSDD

The most frequently cited reasons for not seeking a physician or a sexologist were: *the assumption that HSDD symptoms were normal for their age (35%) and embarrassment (30%)*. The diagnosis of HSDD was often determined by the same physician or sexologist to whom the interviewees initially turned (n = 324). While 21% of women were diagnosed by a gynecologist, symptoms were initially ignored or misdiagnosed by physicians or therapists as depression or anxiety in up to 44% of cases.

Noteworthy: 18% of participants who experienced a delay in diagnosis revealed that their healthcare providers did not know that HSDD was a medical condition, while 13% of these participants felt uncomfortable discussing HSDD as a medical condition.

Regarding the management and treatment of HSDD, patients reported that healthcare providers were much more likely to recommend nonpharmacological treatments. The most commonly recommended were: lubricants, moisturizers (52%), relaxation, meditation, yoga (43%), psychotherapy (39%), weight loss, diet, exercise (32%), and herbal or homeopathic products (19%).

Regardless of the pre or postmenopausal state, patients with HSDD reported that their **relationships with their partners or spouses were most affected**. The sexual elements in the relationship were negatively influenced by HSDD and varied with menopausal status. The overall increase in stress in their relationship was significantly higher among premenopausal women compared to postmenopausal women, and the increase in trust and overall satisfaction was lower among premenopausal women. Consistently, ***participants also reported an increase in the avoidance of situations that could lead to sexual activity***.

Not to mention the effect of HSDD on overall mental well-being.

The study evaluated *the degree of interference in emotional well-being, the ability to "stay in the moment," life satisfaction, being at peace with oneself, feeling happy, sleep quality, positive feelings, mental ability, and the ability to focus on tasks*. The reliability of these endpoints was determined during the pretest evaluation, conducted by sexual medicine experts. Again, *premenopausal women revealed that they were deeply affected in all attributes of overall mental well-being and daily activities* compared to postmenopausal women.

Daily activities included taking care of the partner/spouse, cultivating hobbies, exercising, and spending time with friends, family, and others. ***Regardless of age, participants with HSDD reported that in the past 6 months, they had lost about 11.4 h of work due to HSDD symptoms***. While patients aged between 46 and 60 had been absent from work for about 19.7 hours in the last 6 months.

Finally, they were asked to report the impact of HSDD on their overall life, considering social relationships, mental or emotional well-being, the ability to perform household or personal activities, and work. Responses were evaluated on a scale from 0 to 100, with 0 indicating no interference in any of the factors and 100 indicating maximum interference. Premenopausal patients had significantly higher interference scores compared to postmenopausal women, and women aged between 18 and 45 scored significantly higher than women aged between 46 and 60 and 61 and 80.

It is important to note that fewer than half of patients with sexual problems seek help from doctors or initiate discussions with them. This is due to the fear of shame and the expectation that doctors will initiate such discussions. *When asked about their experience with healthcare providers, women reported that their specialists rarely asked for information about their sexual health.* Certainly, due to clinical experience and specific training on hypoactive sexual desire disorder (HSDD), many doctors refrain from thoroughly investigating the underlying causes of discomfort. The most common statements concern the difficulty of appropriately using the information received from patients and entering an often more sexological field, foreign to their training.

6.3 Pharmacological Therapies: Complications?

Among the most commonly used pharmacological therapies in clinical practice for the treatment of HSDD, **flibanserin** is a treatment approved by the U.S. Food and Drug Administration (FDA) [6]. *This molecule has been shown to induce decreases in serotonin and increases in dopamine and norepinephrine in certain regions of the cerebral cortex* [7].

By modulating these neurotransmitters, it is hypothesized that *flibanserin* restores the balance of excitatory activity [8].

The study by Kornstein SG et al. [9] conducted a retrospective analysis that included data from five studies of the flibanserin clinical development program in HSDD [10].

The research patients included:

- Premenopausal women aged ≥18 years diagnosed with HSDD and enrolled in one of the three randomized, double-blind, placebo-controlled studies evaluating the safety and efficacy of flibanserin [11] (study names: VIOLET, DAISY, BEGONIA).
- Naturally postmenopausal women of any age diagnosed with HSDD and enrolled in a randomized, double-blind, placebo-controlled study to evaluate the safety and efficacy of flibanserin [10] (SNOWDROP).
- Premenopausal women aged ≥18 years who were diagnosed with HSDD and participated in a randomized, placebo-controlled study [12] (VIOLET, DAISY, DAHLIA), a randomized withdrawal study [13] (ROSE), or a pharmacokinetic study of flibanserin and were subsequently enrolled in a 52-week open-label extension study [14] (Sunflower).

The main exclusion criteria included other sexual dysfunctions; major depressive disorder in the past 6 months; history of suicidal ideation or behavior; pelvic inflammatory disease, urinary tract infection, vaginitis, vaginal infection, cervicitis, interstitial cystitis, vulvodynia, or significant vaginal atrophy; ongoing pregnancy or pregnancy in the last month; diagnosis of cancer in the last 10 years; and blood abnormalities.

At the end of 24 weeks, 21.0% of premenopausal women who received *flibanserin* had lost ≥5% of their baseline body weight compared to 7.8% of premenopausal women who received a placebo. Additionally, 3.8% and 2.0% of patients, respectively, experienced a weight loss of ≥10%.

Similarly, 24.7% of postmenopausal women who received *flibanserin* had lost ≥5% of their baseline body weight at week 24, compared to 7.3% of postmenopausal women who received a placebo. Furthermore, 5.2% and 1.7% of patients, respectively, experienced a weight loss of ≥10%. At week 24, a weight gain of ≥7% (the FDA's definition of significant weight gain) was observed in 1.8% and 3.4% of premenopausal women in the *flibanserin* and placebo groups, respectively, and in 2.1% and 2.8% of postmenopausal women, respectively [15].

Among the side effects: nausea, (a common adverse event with flibanserin) was evaluated as a possible factor contributing to weight loss. However, the incidence of nausea in premenopausal women with HSDD who received flibanserin 100 mg in the 24-week randomized placebo-controlled studies *was slightly higher (7.1%) in women with weight loss <5% compared to 5.8% in women with weight loss ≥5%.*

The incidence of nausea was similar in postmenopausal women with weight loss <5% compared to those with weight loss ≥5%, with incidences of 5.3% and 5.6%, respectively.

It should be noted that patients with HSDD recruited in these clinical studies on flibanserin were not selected for overweight or obesity, nor did they enter the studies with the goal of losing weight. In patients with HSDD, the baseline body mass index (BMI) ranged from underweight to obese, with rates of overweight (premenopausal women, 27.2%; postmenopausal women, 34.4%) and obesity (premenopausal women, 24.9%; postmenopausal women, 28.2%) slightly lower than those currently observed in the general population of adult women in the United States [16].

6.4 Bremelanotide: New Drug Approved for the Treatment of HSDD

The study by Mayer D et al. [17] conducted a literature search of *Medline*, *SCOPUS*, and *EMBASE* using the search terms *bremelanotide, bremelanotide injection, Vyleesi* and *melanocortin four receptor agonist* between January 1, 1996, and December 15, 2019. It was found that *bremelanotide* may improve desire and, consequently, lower the level of distress in patients with HSDD. ***However, adverse effects are not lacking: nausea (39.9%), facial flushing (20.4%), and headache (11%).***

Administration: Bremelanotide is a subcutaneous injection that can be administered as needed about 45 minutes before sexual activity. Bremelanotide is safe and has limited pharmacological interactions, including no clinically significant interactions with ethanol. The prescribing guidelines recommend no more than one dose in 24 h and no more than eight doses per month. Individuals should discontinue use after 8 weeks if they do not achieve benefit.

Current treatments for HSDD include psychotherapy and two drugs approved by the U.S. Food and Drug Administration for premenopausal women: **flibanserin**, a mixed serotonin agonist and antagonist, and **bremelanotide**, a melanocortin receptor (MCR) agonist. Melanocortins are endogenous neuropeptides associated with the excitatory pathway of the female sexual response system.

MCRs are found throughout the body, including the brain. *Bremelanotide* is an MCR agonist that non-selectively activates various receptor subtypes, of which subtype 4 (MC4R) is the most relevant at therapeutic doses. MC4R is predominantly expressed in the medial preoptic area (mPOA) of the hypothalamus in the brain and is important for female sexual function. Animal studies suggest that *bremelanotide* may influence female sexual desire by activating presynaptic MC4R on neurons in the hypothalamus's mPOA, leading to an increase in the release of dopamine, an excitatory neurotransmitter that increases sexual desire [18, 19].

6.5 Testosterone for Women Too?

At least 16 million women over the age of 50 currently experience low sexual desire, with about four million women presenting with hypoactive sexual desire disorder (HSDD). Although early research established that testosterone therapy improves sexual desire in postmenopausal women, safer and more effective administration routes have been explored. Large, randomized, double-blind, placebo-controlled studies demonstrate that transdermal testosterone improves sexual function and activity in postmenopausal women with HSDD [20]. More recent studies are exploring the utility of testosterone gels. Although most studies combined testosterone with estrogen or progesterone therapy, the recent ***APHRODITE*** study examined testosterone alone, showing an increase in sexual desire with mild adverse events.

However, some scholars hypothesize an increased risk of breast cancer with the administration of exogenous testosterone. Long-term safety data are now being collected and analyzed, and Phase III studies focusing on long-term risks are underway [21]. The Global Consensus Position Statement on the use of testosterone therapy for women has recommended testosterone therapy for postmenopausal women with HSDD. ***The International Society for the Study of Women's Sexual Health*** appointed a multidisciplinary group of experts who conducted a review of the literature, including original research, meta-analyses, review articles, and consensus guidelines concerning the use of testosterone in women [22]. Although the *Global Position Statement* supports testosterone therapy only for postmenopausal women, limited data also support its use in late reproductive age premenopausal women, in line with the *International Society for the Study of Women's Sexual Health Process of Care for the Management of HSDD*. Systemic transdermal testosterone is recommended for women with HSDD not primarily related to modifiable factors or comorbidities such as relationship or mental health issues. Current research supports a moderate therapeutic benefit. Safety data do not show serious adverse events with the physiological use of testosterone, but long-term safety has not been established. Before starting therapy, physicians must provide informed consent. Shared decision-making involves a full discussion on off-label use, benefits, and risks. A total testosterone level should not be used to diagnose HSDD but as a basis for monitoring. Government-approved male transdermal formulations can be used cautiously with appropriate dosing for women. Patients should be evaluated for signs of androgen excess, and total testosterone levels should be monitored to maintain concentrations within the premenopausal physiological range. This evidence-based guideline is based on a recently published comprehensive meta-analysis and the *Global Position Statement*, approved by numerous societies. The limitation is that testosterone therapy is not approved for women by most regulatory agencies, making prescription and proper dosing difficult. Despite substantial evidence regarding safety, efficacy, and clinical use, access to testosterone therapy for the treatment of HSDD in women remains a significant unmet need [23].

6.6 Conclusions

At the European Society for Sexual Medicine meeting held in Rotterdam in February 2023, several leading experts in the field discussed the multifaceted nature of this disorder and the state of the art in treatment in a roundtable discussion. *HSDD appears to be the most common female sexual disorder, estimated to affect from 28% to 40% of premenopausal women with sexual dysfunction*. **Flibanserin and**

bremelanotide are the only drugs approved for the treatment of HSDD in the United States, and none are approved in Europe. *Lybrido, Lybridos, and Lorexys are in development*. There are several psychological factors that impact sexual desire, including depression and sexual abuse. Evidence strongly supports the value of combining medical and psychological approaches in the treatment of HSDD, but controversy continues regarding the pharmacological treatment of young women with HSDD [19].

The treatment of HSDD, especially in young women, requires a mixed therapeutic approach that addresses the complexity of the pathology. Despite physicians appearing divided between the use of pharmacological and psychosexual approaches, some women may respond better to one type of intervention than to another. *This requires the development of tools that assess the most appropriate approach for each patient, including their willingness and informed choice. In practice, we must ask ourselves "what do women want?"*

Furthermore, the study by Brotto LA et al. [24], reviewing the scientific literature, identified two empirical studies on mindfulness, two on acupuncture, and one on yoga in the treatment of sexual dysfunction.

Mindfulness appears to significantly improve various aspects of sexual response and reduce sexual discomfort in women with sexual desire and arousal disorders. In women with provoked vestibulodynia, acupuncture significantly reduces pain and improves quality of life. There is also case series where acupuncture has significantly improved desire among women with HSDD. Although yoga has only been empirically examined and has proven effective for the treatment of sexual dysfunction (premature ejaculation) in men, numerous historical books cite the benefits of yoga for female sexuality.

Finally, the study by MASEROLI E et al. [25] retrospectively examined a nonselected series of 322 pre- and postmenopausal patients who requested a consultation for FSD. Regular physical activity (measured by frequency: less than 1 hour per week—sedentary; 1–3 h per week—active; 4–6 h per week—very active; more than 6 h per week—extremely active) was studied with a specific question: How helpful can physical activity be in HSDD?

FSD, including HSDD and female genital arousal disorder (FGAD), was diagnosed based on clinical and structured interviews. Participants underwent physical examinations and Doppler ultrasounds of the clitoris completed the Female Sexual Function Index, the Female Sexual Distress Scale-Revised, the Body Uneasiness Test, and the Middlesex Hospital Questionnaire.

In the multivariate analysis, women engaged in physical activity (67.4%) scored significantly higher in several domains of the female sexual function Index, including desire, arousal, and lubrication, and experienced less sexual discomfort and less resistance of the clitoral arteries compared to sedentary women.

A significant inverse association was observed between physical activity and HSDD. *The mediation analysis indicated that the negative association between physical activity and HSDD was partly mediated by concerns about body image (measured by the Body Uneasiness Test), psychopathological symptoms (total score* *of the Middlesex Hospital Questionnaire), and sexual discomfort (score of the Female Sexual Distress Scale-Revised).*

Finally, extreme levels of physical activity were associated with significantly worse scores in several psychosexual parameters including HSDD, sexual satisfaction, and histrionic/hysterical symptoms, even compared to a sedentary lifestyle.

References

1. Shifren JL, Monz BU, Russo PA, Segreti A, Johannes CB. Sexual problems and distress in United States women: prevalence and correlates. Obstet Gynecol. 2008;112:970–8.
2. Nappi RE, Cucinella L, Martella S, Rossi M, Tiranini L, Martini E. Female sexual dysfunction (FSD): prevalence and impact on quality of life (QoL). Maturitas. 2016;94:87–91.
3. Maserejian NN, Parish S, Shifren JL, Huang L, Gerstenberger E, Rosen RC. Healthcare utilization in women diagnosed with hypoactive sexual desire disorder: initial provisional findings from the HSDD registry for women. J Womens Health (Larchmt). 2010;19:2001–9.
4. Parish SJ, Hahn SR. Hypoactive sexual desire disorder: a review of epidemiology, biopsychology, diagnosis, and treatment. Sex Med Rev. 2016;4:103–20.
5. Simon JA, Athavale A, Ravindranath R, Hadker N, Sadiq A, Lim-Watson M, Williams L, Krop J. Assessing the burden of illness associated with acquired generalized hypoactive sexual desire disorder. J Womens Health (Larchmt). 2022;31(5):715–25.
6. Joffe H, Chang C, Sewell C, et al. FDA approval for the Flibanserin: treatment of hypoactive sexual desire disorder. N Engl J Med. 2016;374:101–4.
7. Borsini F, Evans K, Jason K, Rohde F, Alexander B, Pollentier S. Pharmacology of Flibanserin. CNS Drug Rev. 2002;8:117–42.
8. Stahl SM. Sexual desire circuits in hypoactive sexual desire disorder. J Clin Psychiatry. 2010;71:518–9.
9. Kornstein SG, Simon JA, Apfel SC, Yuan J, Barbour KA, Kissling R. Effect of Flibanserin treatment on body weight in premenopausal and postmenopausal women with hypoactive sexual desire disorder: a post hoc analysis. J Womens Health (Larchmt). 2017;26(11):1161–8.
10. Simon JA, Kingsberg SA, Shumel B, Hanes V, Garcia M Jr, Sand M. Efficacy and safety of Flibanserin in postmenopausal women with hypoactive sexual desire disorder: results of the SNOWDROP study. Menopause. 2014;21:633–40.
11. Derogatis LR, Komer L, Katz M, et al. Treatment of hypoactive sexual desire disorder in premenopausal women: efficacy of Flibanserin in the VIOLET study. J Sex Med. 2012;9:1074–85.
12. Thorp J, Simon J, Dattani D, et al. Treatment of hypoactive sexual desire disorder in premenopausal women: efficacy of Flibanserin in the DAISY study. J Sex Med. 2012;9:793–804.
13. Goldfischer ER, Breaux J, Katz M, et al. Continued efficacy and safety of Flibanserin in premenopausal women with hypoactive sexual desire disorder (HSDD): results of a randomized withdrawal study. J Sex Med. 2011;8:3160–72.
14. Jayne C, Simon JA, Taylor LV, Kimura T, Lesko LM. Open-label extension study of Flibanserin in women with hypoactive sexual desire disorder. J Sex Med. 2012;9:3180–8.
15. Sachs GS, Guille C. Weight gain associated with the use of psychotropic medications. J Clin Psychiatry. 1999;60(Suppl 21):16–9.
16. Ogden CL, Carroll MD, Kit BK, Flegal KM. Prevalence of childhood and adult obesity in the United States, 2011–2012. JAMA. 2014;311:806–14.
17. Mayer D, Lynch SE. Bremelanotide: new drug approved for treating hypoactive sexual desire disorder. Ann Pharmacother. 2020;54(7):684–90.
18. Pfaus JG, Sadiq A, Spana C, Clayton AH. The neurobiology of Bremelanotide for the treatment of hypoactive sexual desire disorder in premenopausal women. CNS Spectr. 2022;27(3):281–9.

19. De Oliveira L, Vignozzi L, Giraldi A, Varod S, Corona G, Reisman Y. What women want? The state of the art regarding the treatment of young women with hypoactive sexual desire disorder. Pharmacology. 2024;109(2):69–75.
20. Swanson S, DeRogatis L, Snabes M, Simes S, Zborowski J. Treatment of HSDD in surgically menopausal women: a new phase III, randomized, double-blind, Placebo-controlled, multicenter study on the safety and efficacy of LibiGel. Presented at the annual meeting of the International Society for the Study of women's sexual health, February 22–25, Orlando; 2007.
21. Krapf JM, Simon JA. The role of testosterone in the management of hypoactive sexual desire disorder in postmenopausal women. Maturitas. 2009;63(3):213–9. https://doi.org/10.1016/j.maturitas.2009.04.008. Epub 2009 May 31. PMID: 19487090.
22. Parish SJ, Simon JA, Davis SR, Giraldi A, Goldstein I, Goldstein SW, Kim NN, Kingsberg SA, Morgentaler A, Nappi RE, Park K, Stuenkel CA, Traish AM, Vignozzi L. International Society for the Study of Women's Sexual Health Clinical Practice Guideline for the Use of Systemic Testosterone for Hypoactive Sexual Desire Disorder in Women. J Womens Health (Larchmt). 2021;30(4):474–91. https://doi.org/10.1089/jwh.2021.29037. Epub 2021 Apr 1. PMID: 33797277; PMCID: PMC8064950.
23. Woodis CB, et al. Testosterone supplementation for hypoactive sexual desire disorder in women. Pharmacotherapy. 2012;32(1):38–53.
24. Brotto LA, Krychman M, Jacobson P. Eastern approaches for enhancing women's sexuality: mindfulness, acupuncture, and yoga (CME). J Sex Med. 2008;5(12):2741–8; quiz 2749.
25. Maseroli E, Rastrelli G, Di Stasi V, Cipriani S, Scavello I, Todisco T, Gironi V, Castellini G, Ricca V, Sorbi F, Fambrini M, Petraglia F, Maggi M, Vignozzi L. Physical activity and female sexual dysfunction: a lot helps, but not too much. J Sex Med. 2021;18(7):1217–29.

7 Hypoactive Sexual Desire Disorder and Hypersexuality

Abstract

The concept of "hypersexuality" defines a psychological and behavioral alteration as a result of which sexual stimuli are sought inappropriately, often experienced without desire and intimate satisfaction. This is a psychopathological definition from the scientific community designed to replace terms previously used in other fields of study, such as *nymphomania and satyriasis*, the former referring to females and the latter to males (Bernorio R, Mori G, Casnici F, Polloni G. Diagnostic approach in sexology. Franco Angeli Ed.; Milan, Italy; 2020).

Keywords

Hypoactive desire · Hypersexuality · Nymphomania · Satyriasis · Personality disorders · Bipolar disorder · Sexual arousal · Compulsive behavior · Hypersexual behavior · Hypersexual disorder · Personality assessment · Psychometrics · sexual behavior · *International Classification of Diseases* · ICD-11 · Diagnosis · Complex post-traumatic stress disorder · Prolonged grief disorder · Gambling disorder · Compulsive sexual behavior disorder · Clinical utility · Mental health care

7.1 Introduction

Hypersexuality is included in the two main diagnostic manuals of psychiatric disorders: the *International Classification of Diseases* (ICD) [2] and the *Diagnostic and Statistical Manual of Mental Disorders* (DSM-5-TR) [3]. The ICD is the international classification proposed by the World Health Organization; it is not specific to mental disorders alone, although a section is dedicated to them, and it includes diagnostic criteria for all possible organic disorders. The DSM-5-TR, on the other hand, is a publication by the American Psychiatric Association and is currently the

E. V. Longhi, *Hypoactive Sexual Desire Disorder*,
https://doi.org/10.1007/978-3-032-00659-2_7

most widely used classification in the international scientific community, being entirely dedicated to psychopathologies.

Hypersexuality falls under "Compulsive Sexual Behavior Disorder" in ICD-11, while in DSM-5, it is considered a behavioral addiction that can characterize the pathological conduct of the individual and may also be a dysfunctional trait in other disorders.

The diagnostic criteria advanced by the World Health Organization for hypersexuality are:

A. For at least 6 months, recurrent and intense sexual fantasies, impulses, or behaviors in association with three or more of the following: time spent in repetitive sexual fantasies, impulses, or behaviors that interfere with other important goals, activities, or nonsexual obligations; repetitive involvement in fantasies, impulses, or behaviors in response to dysphoric mood states (such as anxiety, depression, boredom, or irritability); repetitive involvement in fantasies, impulses, or behaviors in response to stressful life events; repeated but unsuccessful efforts to control or significantly reduce such fantasies, impulses, or behaviors; repetitive involvement in sexual behaviors, ignoring the risk of physical or emotional harm to oneself or others.
B. There is clinically significant personal distress or impairment in social, occupational, or other important areas associated with the frequency and intensity of these fantasies, impulses, or behaviors.
C. These fantasies, impulses, or behaviors are not the direct result of medical conditions (such as brain tumors or dementia) or substance use [4].

The study by Montgomery-Graham S et al. [5] evaluated the psychometric qualities of the six most studied HD measurements, including *the Hypersexual Disorder Screening Inventory, the Hypersexual Behavior Inventory, the Sexual Compulsivity Scale, the Sexual Addiction Screening Test, the Sexual Addiction Screening Test-Revised, and the Compulsive Sexual Behavior Inventory.* **Among these**, *the Hypersexual Disorder Screening Inventory* was evaluated as the measurement with the strongest psychometric support.

7.2 Problematic Hypersexuality (PH) and Non-problematic Hypersexuality (NH)

The study by van Tuijl P et al. [6] defined problematic hypersexuality (PH) as the experience of discomfort and negative consequences due to hypersexual impulses and behaviors, to the extent that it leads the individual to seek help. Meanwhile, non-problematic hypersexuality (NH) describes those who experience high levels of sexual desire but without the associated discomfort [7].

Reviewing the literature, however, one could argue that the concept of hypersexuality itself is too broad and does not apply exclusively to pathological hypotheses.

We know that hypersexuality becomes pathological:

(a) When the individual experiences clinically significant distress related to their sexual conduct, which does not always coincide with internal discomfort in realizing their own drives but depends on the social judgment of the community in which they live—be it the couple, friends, family, work, or social nucleus.
(b) When the individual exhibits a significant and disproportionate increase in sexual drive for at least 6 months, which does not always correspond to the satisfaction of sexual desire and consists of recurring and intrusive fantasies and thoughts, excessive sexual behaviors, and an inability to control their own sexuality, despite negative consequences.
(c) When the individual, in realizing their sexual drives, engages in paraphilic dysfunctional behaviors, either in comorbidity with them or with sexual dysfunctions [8, 9].

For this reason, the *Perrotta Hypersexuality Global Spectrum of Gradation* **(PH-GSS)** is proposed, which distinguishes high-functioning forms—proactive and dynamic hypersexuality—from those with attenuated and impaired functioning—dysfunctional and pathological hypersexuality of grades I and II—is suggested. Hypersexuality, therefore, is a potentially clinically relevant condition, consisting of one or more dysfunctional and pathological behaviors related to an individual's sexual sphere, which can be explained more consistently and reproducibly according to the neurobiological theoretical model.

7.3 Psychometric Scales

Most scales related to hypersexuality contain a factor that evaluates the negative consequences of hypersexuality. One of the most frequently used self-reported assessments, the hypersexual behavior inventory, consists of three subscales, including the four-item consequences subscale, for example: "My sexual thoughts and fantasies distract me from completing important tasks" [10].

The Sexual Addiction Screening Test-Revised (SAST-R) has two factors related to the outcome [11]:

1. The relationship disturbance factor, which consists of items on conflicts and interpersonal difficulties, such as: "Has your sexual behavior ever caused problems for you and your family?"
2. The affect disturbance factor, which includes questions about intrapersonal problems, such as: "Do you ever feel bad about your sexual behavior?"

Although the compulsive sexual behavior inventory does not contain an entire factor dedicated to negative consequences, it introduces elements that evaluate problems related to sexual behavior in financial, relational, and emotional areas:

"How often have your sexual activities caused you financial problems?" or "How often have you felt guilty or embarrassed about aspects of your behavior?" [12].

A more recent scale to measure hypersexuality is the Compulsive Sexual Behavior Disorder Scale (CSBD-19), which also contains a factor dedicated to negative consequences: "My sexual activities have interfered with my work and/or my education" or "I have often found myself in an embarrassing situation because of my sexual behavior" [13].

The disorder of **compulsive sexual behavior (CSBD)**, also known as sex addiction, hypersexual disorder, hypersexuality, sexual compulsivity, sexual impulsivity, or out-of-control sexual behaviors, is included in the 11th revision of the *International Classification of Diseases (ICD-11)*.

For a diagnosis of CSBD, these sexual behaviors must cause *clinically significant distress, neglect of responsibilities, interests, and health, and result in significant impairment in critical areas of functioning*. In particular, people with CSBD derive little or no satisfaction from their sexual activities and often make unsuccessful efforts to reduce or stop their behavior.

So far, only a few studies have examined the prevalence of CSBD among nationally representative samples, all of which have been conducted in the United States, Germany, Hungary, and Poland. Based on the results of these studies, ***3–10% of men and 2–7% of women may experience CSBD***.

In particular, the study by Bőthe B et al. [14] ***used the International Sex Survey (ISS) in 42 countries, in 26 languages.***

A total of 82,243 participants were recruited, with an average age of 32.39 years. Most of the participants were women (57.0%), followed by men (39.6%) and individuals of different genders (3.4%). Most participants were heterosexual (68.2%), while 31.5% identified as sexually diverse (i.e., used terms other than heterosexual to describe their sexual orientation). Most of the participants held a degree (74.0%) and worked full time (52.3%).

The highest CSBD scores were observed in Turkey, followed by China and Peru. All pairwise comparisons between countries revealed pathological dimensions ranging from minimal to moderate. Men scored highest on the CSBD-19, followed by individuals of different genders and women, with a moderate pathological dimension. No differences based on sexual orientation were observed when comparing the eight groups by sexual orientation.

Moreover, the high-risk group reported significantly higher levels of solitary sexual activity (autoeroticism) and couple partnered activity (sexual activity with a casual partners) compared to the low risk group. Of the high-risk group, 13.7% had previously sought treatment for CSBD, with an additional 32.8% who had not sought treatment primarily for economic reasons. Only 1.6% of the low-risk group had never sought treatment for CSBD, and 3.3% excluded treatment for various reasons (social, religious, etc.). ***In conclusion, with a global incidence rate of nearly 5%, CSBD appears to be as widespread as other more extensively studied psychiatric disorders***. The study by Reed GM et al. [15] focused on four core CSBD disorders: *complex post-traumatic stress disorder, prolonged grief disorder, gambling disorder, and compulsive sexual behavior disorder, as defined in ICD-11.*

Among the significant changes in the *ICD-11* is the addition of 21 new mental disorders. These new categories are generally proposed to: (a) improve the utility of morbidity statistics; (b) facilitate the recognition of clinically significant but poorly classified mental disorders, thereby providing appropriate management; and (c) stimulate research on more effective treatments. The 11th revision of the *International Classification of Diseases (ICD-11)* by the *World Health Organization (WHO)* was approved by the World Health Assembly—composed of health ministers from all WHO member states—on May 25, 2019. Reporting health statistics based on this new diagnostic system commenced on January 1, 2022 [16]. WHO member states are transitioning from ICD-10 to ICD-11, a process expected to take several years to achieve fully global implementation. Countries that have not yet implemented ICD-11 in their health information and reporting systems will use conversion algorithms to comply with WHO reporting requirements in the meantime. *Over the past 10 years, in the context of the overall development of ICD-11, the WHO Department of Mental Health and Substance Use have developed Clinical Descriptions and Diagnostic Requirements (CDDR) for ICD-11 Mental, Behavioral and Neurodevelopmental Disorders*, aiming to provide sufficient information for reliable clinical implementation. The development of the ICD-11 CDDR, based on principles of clinical utility and global applicability, was the most extensive, multilingual, multidisciplinary, and participatory revision process ever undertaken for a classification of mental disorders [17].

7.4 Hypersexuality and Couple Relationships in Bipolar Disorder

Although changes in sexual behavior are recognized as an integral part of bipolar disorder, most of the relevant literature on sexual problems in patients with this condition concerns medication side effects and does not differentiate bipolar disorder from other severe mental disorders. The study by Kopeykina I et al. [18] used ***PsycINFO and PubMed*** with keywords related to bipolar disorder, hypersexuality, and couple relationships. A total of 27 articles were selected. The literature indicates a higher incidence of risky sexual behaviors in bipolar patients during manic episodes compared to patients with other psychiatric diagnoses. Furthermore, studies examining sexuality in couples with a bipolar partner found reduced levels of sexual satisfaction associated with the diagnosis, a higher incidence of sexual dysfunction during depressive episodes, and disparate levels of overall satisfaction between patients and their partners. Finally, although bipolar patients experience specific sexual problems related to mania-induced hypersexuality and specific effects of mood cycles on couple relationships, the literature often lacks a consistent definition of hypersexuality. Severe impulse control disorders involving **pathological gambling, hypersexuality, and compulsive shopping** have been reported in association with the use of dopamine receptor agonist drugs in a series of retrospective patient surveys. *These agents are also used to treat Parkinson's disease, restless leg syndrome, and hyperprolactinemia.* A retrospective disproportionality analysis was conducted based on the 2.7 million reports of serious adverse drug events, both domestic and foreign, from 2003 to 2012, extracted from the *Food and Drug Administration* (FDA) *Adverse Event Reporting System* [19].

Cases were selected if they contained any of the ten preferred terms in the *Medical Dictionary for Regulatory Activities* (MedDRA) that described abnormal behaviors.

A total of **1580** events indicating impulse control disorders were identified from the United States and 21 other countries: 710 for dopamine receptor agonist drugs and 870 for other medications. Dopamine receptor agonist drugs showed a strong signal associated with these impulse control disorders. The association was strongest for the dopamine agonist pramipexole, which has a preferential affinity for the dopamine D3 receptor. A signal was also observed for aripiprazole, an antipsychotic classified as a partial agonist of the D3 receptor.

7.5 What Do We Mean by Hypersexuality in Children and Adolescents?

Psychiatric literature has used the term "hypersexuality" to indicate pathologically increased sexual behavior in children and adolescents. *Various patterns of increased sexuality in young people have been described, including excessive, developmentally precocious, compulsive, aggressive, or otherwise socially inappropriate sexuality*. This "hypersexual" behavior in children and adolescents is associated with a variety of factors.

Social factors include sexual abuse, physical abuse, life stress, and compromised family relationships. Psychiatric factors include general emotional and behavioral problems, post-traumatic stress disorder, dissociative symptoms in particular, and possibly bipolar disorder.

Despite the importance of increased sexual behavior in young people as a possible sign of these problems, there is currently no uniform definition in psychiatric literature of the term "hypersexuality" as applied to children and adolescents. The utility of this term depends on the extent to which it can be defined, measured, and distinguished from non-pathological youthful sexual behavior.

Research tools are described that can be useful for measuring levels of sexual behavior in children and adolescents. Elements of a definition of youthful hypersexuality are proposed based on current knowledge about the sexuality of children and adolescents in both normal development and a variety of conditions where it is increased. Care is justified in distinguishing between normal and abnormal sexual behavior in young people because of the variety of factors that can influence its measurement [20].

Excessive sexual behavior has also been reported in young people who may be affected by *Juvenile Bipolar Disorder (JBD)* and has been termed "hypersexuality". Although there is no universal definition of this term, this observation has led to a hypothesis that *increased sexual behavior characterizes bipolar syndrome in children and adolescents and differentiates it from attention deficit hyperactivity disorder.*

Although this hypothesis is plausible, the supporting evidence is incomplete. Moreover, studies to test it should control for factors other than JBD that are known to increase sexual behavior in children and adolescents. These include related sexual abuse, post-traumatic stress disorder, excessive exposure to sexual stimuli, general psychiatric illness, and social variables such as family chaos and social stress. Some of these factors may increase sexual behavior in young people with bipolar disorder through psychodynamic mechanisms rather than as a result of the disease itself. Therefore, further research is needed to determine whether hyperactive sexual behavior can serve as a diagnostic criterion for bipolar disorder in children and adolescents.

7.6 Hypersexuality, ADHD, Hypersexuality and Paraphilias

Individuals with ADHD suffer from inattention, hyperactivity, and impulsivity. Doctors often assume that specific ADHD symptoms influence sexual desire by increasing the frequency of hypersexuality. There is a lack of knowledge regarding the comorbidity between ADHD, hypersexuality, and paraphilias. The study by Soldati L et al. [21] provided a review of the literature on the association of ADHD, hypersexuality, and paraphilias discussing the screening for and management of these conditions when associated with ADHD. A systematic review of the literature was performed in the databases *PubMed, PsychInfo, and Embase.*

The studies examined show that some individuals suffering from ADHD report hypersexuality and paraphilias, but no clear data emerged to support the idea that hypersexuality and paraphilias are more frequent in a population with ADHD. On the other hand, some studies have shown a high prevalence of ADHD in hypersexual and paraphilic subjects. This is the first systematic review of hypersexuality and paraphilias in individuals with ADHD. However, the results are limited by the small number of studies and the small sample sizes of many of the included research.

In the study by **Bőthe B et al.** [22] a multigroup structural equation modeling was conducted to investigate the hypothesized associations between adult ADHD symptoms, hypersexuality, and problematic pornography use (PPU) among men and women (N = 14,043 participants; women = 4237; average age = 33.5 years, SD = 10.9).

The symptoms of ADHD in adults were evaluated concerning hypersexuality and PPU through self-reported measures. The results indicated that *hypersexuality had a positive, moderate association with problematic pornography use among women and a very significant association among men.* The symptoms of ADHD had positive, moderate associations with hypersexuality in both men and women. Regarding men, ADHD symptoms had a positive, moderate association with PPU, while in women; ADHD symptoms had a weak association with PPU.

In conclusion, *ADHD symptoms could play an important role in the severity of hypersexuality in both sexes, while they may play a more significant role in PPU only among men.*

The results support previous findings that PPU may not be unequivocally considered a subcategory of hypersexuality. Furthermore, the potential underlying mechanisms of problematic pornography use should be examined separately in men and women.

Previous research has identified some peculiarities in the sexual functioning of adults with ADHD. Using online questionnaires, the study by Turner D et al. [23] evaluated the prevalence of paraphilic fantasies and behaviors in a sample of **160** adults with ADHD compared to 75 adults without ADHD, examining the association between paraphilias and hypersexuality in the ADHD group.

Both groups reported high rates of paraphilic fantasies and behaviors. *Individuals with ADHD were more likely to report sexually exciting paraphilic fantasies and behaviors*. Additionally, individuals with ADHD reported, on average, more sexually exciting paraphilic behaviors than those without ADHD. In patients with ADHD, sexually exciting paraphilic interests in masturbation fantasies and sexual behaviors showed a significant correlation with hypersexuality.

No significant correlation was found in individuals without ADHD. *Overall, it can be concluded that individuals with ADHD are more prone to develop and enact paraphilic sexuality compared to those without ADHD; however, the differences found were minimal.*

7.7 Conclusions

Hypersexuality appears to be a complex pathology that requires specific history taking and further research. An example of this is the limited number of studies examining the *clinical characteristics of post-September 11 U.S. military veterans dealing with alcohol problems*.

In particular, the research by Moisson J et al. [24] examined psychopathology and hypersexuality among male and female post-September 11 veterans with and without a history of alcohol use disorder (AUD).

Data obtained via telephone interviews from a national convenience sample of **283** U.S. veterans were analyzed. Many of them (39.1%) met criteria for lifetime AUD. It was also found that veterans with lifetime AUD met clinically significant levels of post-traumatic stress disorder and criteria for drug use disorders (lifetime). Veterans with lifetime AUD attended religious services less often, engaged in more solitary self-erotic experiences in the previous month, and reported problematic use of pornography and hypersexuality compared to veterans without AUD. Logistic regression analysis identified lifetime drug use disorders and symptoms of post-traumatic stress disorder as significant predictors of lifetime AUD status.

References

1. Bernorio R., Mori G., Casnici F., Polloni G. Diagnostic approach in sexology. Franco Angeli Ed.; Milan, Italy: 2020.
2. World Health Organization (WHO) ICD-11: International Classification of Diseases, 11th Revision; 2022. [(consulted on March 30, 2023)]. Available online: https://icd.who.int/ [Reference list].
3. American Psychiatric Association (APA). Diagnostic and statistical manual of mental disorders. 5th ed. Washington, DC: American Psychiatric Association; 2013.
4. Montgomery-Graham S. Conceptualization and evaluation of hypersexual disorder: a systematic review of the literature. Sex Med Rev. 2017;5:146–62. https://doi.org/10.1016/j.sxmr.2016.11.001.
5. Montgomery-Graham S. Conceptualization and assessment of hypersexual disorder: a systematic review of the literature. Sex Med Rev. 2017;5(2):146–62. https://doi.org/10.1016/j.sxmr.2016.11.001. Epub 2016 Dec 29. PMID: 28041854.
6. van Tuijl P, Verboon P, van Lankveld J. Initial development and validation of item banks to measure problematic hypersexuality. Open Res Eur. 2024;3:129. https://doi.org/10.12688/openreseurope.16131.2. PMID: 39118807; PMCID: PMC11306953.
7. Briken P, Wiessner C, Štulhofer A, et al. Who feels affected by "out of control" sexual behavior? Prevalence and correlates of indicators for compulsive sexual behavior disorder ICD-11 in the German health and sexuality survey (GeSiD). J Behav Addict. 2022;11(3):900–11.
8. Parra-Dìaz P, Chico-Garcìa JL, Beltràn-Corbellini A, Rodrìguez-Jorge F, Fernàndez-Escandòn CL, Alonso-Cànovas A, Martìnez-Castrillo JC. Does the country make a difference in impulse control disorders? A systematic review. Mov Disorder Clin Pract. 2020;8:25–32.
9. Perrotta G. Dysfunctional sexual behaviors: definition, clinical contexts, neurobiological profiles and treatments. Int J Sex Reprod Health Care. 2020;3:61–9.
10. Reid RC, Carpenter BN, Hook JN, Garos S, Manning JC, Gilliland R, et al. Report of the results of a field trial of the DSM-5 for hypersexual disorder. J Sex Med. 2012;9(11):2868–77.
11. Carnes PJ, Green BA, Merlo LJ, Polles A, Carnes S. Gold MS PATHOS: a brief screening application for the evaluation of sexual addiction. J Addict Med. 2012;6(1):29.
12. Coleman E, Miner M, Ohlerking F, Raymond NE. Compulsive sexual behavior inventory: a preliminary study of reliability and validity. J Sex Marital Ther. 2001;27(4):325–32.
13. Bőthe B, Potenza MN, Griffiths MD, Kraus SW, Klein V, Fuss J, Demetrovics ZS. The development of the compulsive sexual behavior disorder scale (CSBD-19): an ICD-11 based screening measure in three languages. J Behav Addict. 2020; https://doi.org/10.1556/2006.2020.00034.
14. Bőthe B, Koós M, Nagy L, Kraus SW, Demetrovics Z, Potenza MN, Michaud A, Ballester-Arnal R, Batthyány D, Bergeron S, Billieux J, Briken P, Burkauskas J, Cárdenas-López G, Carvalho J, Castro-Calvo J, Chen L, Ciocca G, Corazza O, Csako R, Fernandez DP, Fernandez EF, Fournier L, Fujiwara H, Fuss J, Gabrhelík R, Gewirtz-Meydan A, Gjoneska B, Gola M, Grubbs JB, Hashim HT, Islam MS, Ismail M, Jiménez-Martínez MC, Jurin T, Kalina O, Klein V, Költő A, Lee CT, Lee SK, Lewczuk K, Lin CY, Liverpool John Moores University's research team, Lochner C, López-Alvarado S, Lukavská K, Mayta-Tristán P, Milea I, Miller DJ, Orosová O, Orosz G, Sungkyunkwan University's Research Team, Ponce FP, Quintana GR, Quintero Garzola GC, Ramos-Diaz J, Rigaud K, Rousseau A, De Tubino Scanavino M, Schulmeyer MK, Sharan P, Shibata M, Shoib S, Sigre Leirós VL, Sniewski L, Spasovski O, Steibliene V, Stein DJ, Strizek J, Štulhofer A, Ünsal BC, Vaillancourt-Morel MP. Compulsive sexual behavior disorder in 42 countries: insights from the international sex survey and introduction of standardized assessment tools. J Behav Addict. 2023;12(2):393–407. https://doi.org/10.1556/2006.2023.00028. PMID: 37352095; PMCID: PMC10316175.
15. Reed GM, First MB, Billieux J, Cloitre M, Briken P, Achab S, Brewin CR, King DL, Kraus SW, Bryant RA. Emerging experience with selected new categories in the ICD-11: complex PTSD, prolonged grief disorder, gaming disorder, and compulsive sexual behaviour disorder. World Psychiatry. 2022;21(2):189–213. https://doi.org/10.1002/wps.20960. PMID: 35524599; PMCID: PMC9077619.

16. World Health Organization. International Statistical Classification of Diseases and Related Health Problems. https://www.who.int.
17. Reed GM, First MB, Kogan CS, et al. Innovations and changes in the ICD-11 classification of mental, behavioral and neurodevelopmental disorders. World Psychiatry. 2019;18:3–19.
18. Kopeykina I, Kim HJ, Khatun T, Boland J, Haeri S, Cohen LJ, Galynker II. Hypersexuality and couple relationships in bipolar disorder: a review. J Affect Disord. 2016;195:1–14.
19. Moore TJ, Glenmullen J, Mattison DR. Reports of pathological gambling, hypersexuality, and compulsive shopping associated with dopamine receptor agonist drugs. JAMA Intern Med. 2014;174(12):1930–3.
20. Adelson S, Bell R, Graff A, Goldenberg D, Haase E, Downey JI, Friedman RC. Toward a definition of "hypersexuality" in children and adolescents. Psychodyn Psychiatry. 2012;40(3):481–503. https://doi.org/10.1521/pdps.2012.40.3.481. PMID: 23002706.
21. Soldati L, Bianchi-Demicheli F, Schockaert P, Köhl J, Bolmont M, Hasler R, Perroud N. Association of ADHD and hypersexuality and paraphilias. Psychiatry Res. 2021;295:113638. https://doi.org/10.1016/j.psychres.2020.113638. Epub 2020 Dec 10. PMID: 33333439.
22. Bőthe B, Koós M, Tóth-Király I, Orosz G, Demetrovics Z. Investigating the associations of adult ADHD symptoms, hypersexuality, and problematic pornography use among men and women on a largescale, non-clinical sample. J Sex Med. 2019;16(4):489–99. https://doi.org/10.1016/j.jsxm.2019.01.312. Epub 2019 Mar 7. PMID: 30852107.
23. Turner D, Gregório Hertz P, Biedermann L, Barra S, Retz W. Paraphilic fantasies and behavior in attention deficit/hyperactivity disorder and their association with hypersexuality. Int J Impot Res. 2024; https://doi.org/10.1038/s41443-024-00891-w. Epub ahead of print. PMID: 38637719.
24. Moisson J, Potenza MN, Shirk SD, Hoff RA, Park CL, Kraus SW. Psychopathology and hypersexuality among veterans with and without histories of alcohol-use disorders. Am J Addict. 2019;28(5):398–404. https://doi.org/10.1111/ajad.12941. Epub 2019 Aug 8. PMID: 31393652.

Part III

Psychosocial and Relational Dimensions

Partner Responses in Couples Coping with HSDD

8

Abstract

Sexual dysfunctions are widespread, affecting approximately 43% of women and 31% of men. ***Hypoactive sexual desire disorder has been reported in about 30% of women and 15% of men in population-based studies and is associated with a wide variety of medical and psychological causes***. Sexual arousal disorders, including erectile dysfunction in men and female sexual arousal disorder in women, are found in 10–20% of men and women and are strongly correlated with age in men. Orgasmic disorder is relatively common in women and affects about 10%–15% in community-based studies. Conversely, premature ejaculation is the most common sexual disorder in men, with a reporting rate of about 30% in most studies. Finally, sexual pain disorders have been reported in 10%–15% of women and less than 5% of men. In addition to their widespread prevalence, it has been found that sexual dysfunctions have a significant impact on interpersonal functioning and overall quality of life in both men and women (Rosen RC, Curr Psychiatry Rep 2(3):189–195, 2000).

Keywords

HSDD · Couples · Female pathologies underlying HSDD · Partner responses · FSIAD

8.1 Introduction

When symptoms of low sexual desire in men persist for at least 6 months, they cause clinically significant distress for themselves and their partners. The DSM-5 diagnosis of hypoactive sexual desire disorder takes into account male patients, including transgender, intersex, and queer individuals.

E. V. Longhi, *Hypoactive Sexual Desire Disorder*,
https://doi.org/10.1007/978-3-032-00659-2_8

However, it is estimated that the prevalence rates of hypoactive sexual desire disorder (HSDD) range from 1% to 20% in men, varying according to the evaluation method, the age of the sample, and the country [2].

A population-based study in the United Kingdom revealed that 14.9% of nearly 5000 men had experienced low desire for at least 3 months of the previous year. These high rates of low desire are concerning; low sexual desire has been linked to increased depression and stress, lower sexual satisfaction, lower relationship satisfaction and quality, and disruption of other aspects of sexual function, such as erectile function [3].

8.2 Natsal 3

The study by Mitchell KR et al. [3], named Natsal-3, was a survey of 15,162 men and women aged between 16 and 74 years in Great Britain (England, Scotland, and Wales). The interviews took place between September 6, 2010, and August 31, 2012. The estimated response rate was 57.7%, and the cooperation rate was estimated at 65.8%. Participants completed the survey through a combination of computer-assisted face-to-face interviews, as well as self-interviews.

Natsal-3 was born from a collaboration between University College London (London, UK), *London School of Hygiene & Tropical Medicine* (London, UK), NatCen Social Research, Public Health England (formerly the Health Protection Agency), and the University of Manchester (Manchester, UK). The study was supported by grants from the Medical Research Council (G0701757) and the Wellcome Trust (084840), with contributions from the Economic and Social Research Council and the Department of Health. NF is funded by a National Institute for Health Research (NIHR) Academic Clinical Lectureship.

The research concluded that patients most likely to have low sexual function were those *without a steady partner*, similar to those who *had ended a relationship*. Furthermore, patients who were not satisfied with their relationship were more likely to have low sexual function, as well as *finding it difficult to talk about sex with their partner*. Low sexual functionality was also associated with a lack of sexual competence at first intercourse and with a *low frequency of sexual activity, often replaced by masturbation* [4].

The British study also highlighted an association between low sexual function and having had *a same-sex partner in the last 5 years*. For men, an association was reported between low sexual functionality and paid sexual intercourse in the past year. Women reported a greater number of sexual partners in their intimate experiences. HSDD was also associated with negative sexual experiences or sexual intercourse with outcomes of sexually transmitted diseases in the past 5 years.

The study also highlighted that the most commonly reported problems by **men** were lack of interest in sex (14.9%), premature ejaculation (14.9%), and erectile dysfunction (12.9%). For **women**, the most common problems were lack of interest in sex (34.2%), difficulty reaching orgasm (16.3%), vaginal dryness (13.0%), and absence of pleasure (12.1%). Lack of interest was twice as common among women compared to men. In younger participants, aged between 16 and 24, the most common problem among men was premature ejaculation (16.5%); in women, it was lack of interest in sex (24.8%) and difficulty reaching orgasm (21.0%).

8.3 Most Common Partner Responses

Other scientific research has identified three distinct partner responses to sexual difficulties [5]:

- Positive or facilitating responses (affectionate, empathetic)
- Negative responses (hostile, critical) and
- Solicitous responses (overly understanding or avoiding).

This suggests that, in the face of sexual dysfunction—which is often stressful—the positive or facilitating responses of partners encourage problem resolution or help-seeking from a sexologist. Both partners derived greater sexual well-being from this. Conversely, negative responses promote less adaptive strategies, such as avoidance or emotional suppression, ultimately contributing to lower sexual well-being [6].

The studies of Rosen NO et al. [6] also highlighted that in patients with vulvodynia suffering from HSDD, associated with painful intercourse, the following responses are elicited in partners:

- Attention and sympathy
- In negative cases, hostility and frustration
- Facilitating responses (encouragement of adaptation).

No research has evaluated the influence of daily partner responses in this population. Moreover, there is limited knowledge about the impact of partner responses on sexual function, which is a consequence of the partner's sexual impairment.

Similarly, patients who report HSDD resulting from provoked vestibulodynia (PVD) experience recurrent vulvovaginal pain, primarily triggered during sexual intercourse, and a permanent absence of sexual desire. Although affected couples report negative effects on their overall sexual and romantic relationships, few studies have examined the interpersonal factors that may influence their sexual and relational satisfaction. Cross-sectional studies have shown that greater caring and negative partner responses and fewer facilitating responses are associated with lower sexual and relational satisfaction in women with PVD-related HSDD [7].

There is no doubt that the partner's response is therapeutic in the partial or total overcoming of HSDD. The couple's relationship style—whether complicity, conflict, symbiosis, or judgment—is at the basis of mutual motivation and, consequently, of sexual desire and the frequency of intercourse.

In fact, the experience of HSDD or distressing sexual arousal (Feminine Sexual Interest/Arousal Disorder, FSIAD) is prevalent in women of all ages and is associated with lower sexual, relational, and psychological well-being compared to women without this difficulty. Women who have a partner report almost five times more likely to be distressed by low desire and to receive a diagnosis of FSIAD compared to women without a partner, indicating that interpersonal factors are highly relevant, although largely overlooked in past research.

Scientific research is unanimous: when women with FSIAD perceive more positive partner responses—warm, supportive, and compassionate—compared to negative responses—hostile, unsupportive, and indifferent—they are more satisfied with the relationship, and both they and their partners report lower anxiety. When partners report more positive than negative responses, they have greater sexual and relational satisfaction, as well as less sexual discomfort and anxiety. Exploratory analyses have revealed that women's perceptions of their partners' responses explain the link between partner responses and women's relationship satisfaction and anxiety. Partner responses did not predict any change in outcomes over time [8].

There are still unclear points. Women diagnosed with female sexual interest/arousal disorder (FSIAD) report lower health-related quality of life, more depressive symptoms, and less sexual and relational satisfaction compared to healthy control subjects. Despite the impact of HSDD and FSIAD on female sexuality, and the inherently interpersonal nature of the sexual problem, it is still unclear whether the partners of women with FSIAD face consequent sexual dysfunctions.

The study by NO Rosen, et al. [9], recruited **97 patients** diagnosed with HSDD and FSIAD and their respective partners ($n = 97$) and **108 couples** for the control group. All recruited patients independently completed questionnaires related to sexual desire, sexual discomfort, sexual function, sexual satisfaction, sexual communication, relational satisfaction, depression, and anxiety.

The partners of women with FSIAD reported lower sexual satisfaction, poorer sexual communication, and greater sexual discomfort, compared to control partners. The male partners of women with FSIAD reported greater difficulties with orgasmic and erectile functioning, and less overall satisfaction and sexual intercourse satisfaction on the International Index of Erectile Function (IIEF), compared to control partners.

Women with hypoactive sexual desire disorder HSDD and FSIAD reported less desire and sexual satisfaction, and greater sexual discomfort, and more depressive and anxiety symptoms compared to both control women and their own partners. They also reported poorer sexual communication compared to control women. Women with HSDD and FSIAD also reported less sexual desire, arousal, lubrication, and satisfaction, and more pain during sexual intercourse on the Female Sexual Function Index (FSFI), compared to control women.

The study by Elisa Maseroli et al. [10] recruited **133** women who sought a specialist for HSDD and were evaluated for clinical, biochemical, and psychosexual data at the first visit. A group of **55** patients with HSDD treated for 6 months with transdermal testosterone was then analyzed. The *Sexual Inhibition Scale* (SIS) and *Sexual Excitation Scale* (SES) questionnaires were used.

Patients with altered SIS scores showed greater suffering and psychopathological symptoms, while those with altered SES scores demonstrated a desire and arousal lower than the norm, with altered metabolic and hormonal parameters. The SES score also showed a significant effect on the effectiveness of testosterone treatment for HSDD.

8.4 Conclusions

The investigation and therapy for HSDD predisposes to a transdisciplinary approach, which implies not only the collaboration of multidisciplinary professionals but also the review of practices, clinical and research, to ensure the highest level of care provided.

Studies have consistently demonstrated *the interdependence of sexual function between partners, with dysfunction in one partner often contributing to problems in sexual functioning and/or sexual satisfaction for the other*. It is essential that clinicians *explore patients' attachment styles, childhood experiences (including sexual abuse), the onset of sexual activity, personality, cognitive patterns, infertility problems, and sexual expectations*. The evaluation of depression, anxiety, stress, substance use, and post-traumatic stress should be part of the first visit; even if anxiety and/or depression seem a consequence or a cause of the sexual disorder. Also, *cognitive distraction* is a significant factor contributing to sexual response problems in men and women and is observed more consistently for genital arousal than for subjective arousal. To these factors is added the evaluation of organic and mental diseases, whether incidental or hereditary. Lastly, extensive psychosexual support for HSDD and difficulties in orgasm in women and men, where possible, is highlighted.

References

1. American Psychiatric Association. Diagnostic and statistical manual of mental disorders, 5th ed. American Psychiatric Press; 2013. Rosen RC. Prevalence and risk factors of sexual dysfunction in men and women. Curr Psychiatry Rep. 2000;2(3):189–95. https://doi.org/10.1007/s11920-996-0006-2.
2. Brotto LA. DSM diagnostic criteria for hypoactive sexual desire disorder in men. J Sex Med. 2010;7(5):2015–30.
3. Mitchell KR, Mercer CH, Ploubidis GB, et al. Sexual function in Britain: findings from the third National Survey of Sexual Attitudes and Lifestyles (Natsal-3). Lancet. 2013;382(9907):1817–29.
4. Wellings K, Nanchahal K, Macdowall W. Sexual behavior in Britain: early heterosexual experience. Lancet. 2001;358:1843–50.
5. Rosen NO, Bergeron S. Genito-pelvic pain through a dyadic lens: towards a model of interpersonal emotion regulation of female sexual dysfunction. J Sex Res. 2019;56(4–5):440–61.
6. Rosen NO, Bergeron S, Sadikaj G, Glowacka M, Delisle I, Baxter ML. Impact of male partner responses on sexual function in women with vulvodynia and their partners: a dyadic daily experience study. Health Psychol. 2014;33(8):823–31.
7. Rosen NO, Muise A, Bergeron S, Delisle I, Baxter ML. Daily associations between partner responses and sexual and relationship satisfaction in couples coping with provoked Vestibulodynia. J Sex Med. 2015;12(4):1028–39. https://doi.org/10.1111/jsm.12840.

8. Rosen NO, Corsini-Munt S, Dubé JP, Boudreau C, Muise A. Partner responses to low desire: associations with sexual, relationship, and psychological Well-being among couples coping with female sexual interest/arousal disorder. J Sex Med. 2020;17(11):2168–80. https://doi.org/10.1016/j.jsxm.2020.08.015.
9. Rosen NO, Dubé JP, Corsini-Munt S, Muise A. Partners also experience consequences: a comparison of the sexual, relationship, and psychological adjustment of women with female sexual interest/arousal disorder and their partners to control couples. J Sex Med. 2019;16(1):83–95. https://doi.org/10.1016/j.jsxm.2018.10.018.
10. Maseroli E, Cipriani S, Lanzi V, Ravelli SA, Annunziato M, Alfaroli C, Lippi D, Cirillo M, Castellini G, Giraldi A, Maggi M, Vignozzi L. Hypoactive sexual desire disorder in women: new possibilities for ensuring a better understanding, diagnosis, and response to treatment. J Sex Med. 2024;21(10):861–71. https://doi.org/10.1093/jsxmed/qdae102.

HSDD and Body Image

9

Abstract

Numerous studies confirm that body image influences multiple aspects of an individual's psychosocial, relational, psychological, and sexual functioning, in both men and women. One of the potential concerns related to body image (BI) is the lack of sexual appeal. Body image is often described as how a person perceives their own body to be more or less suitable to seduce and/or appear seductive to the surrounding world.

Keywords

Body image · Hypoactive sexual desire disorder · Quality of life · Eating disorders · Adolescence and inadequate body image · Motherhood and body inadequacy

9.1 Introduction

Various factors can influence variations and fluctuations in sexual desire, including biological and psychosexual factors related to the social context [1]. One of the psychological factors associated with hypoactive sexual desire disorder (HSDD) may be concern about urinary incontinence. Body image, or in other words, the mental image of the body, represents the way individuals think, feel, and behave about their physical attributes [2]. It has been conceptualized as a complex and multidimensional construct capable of influencing quality of life, as well as affective, cognitive, and behavioral functioning.

The study by Cash TF et al. [3] stated that body image includes three dimensions: evaluation, investment, and affect. Body image evaluation defines feelings of satisfaction or dissatisfaction towards one's appearance. Investment in body image refers to the importance attributed to physical appearance and the effort one is

E. V. Longhi, *Hypoactive Sexual Desire Disorder*,
https://doi.org/10.1007/978-3-032-00659-2_9

willing to invest to achieve the desired physical appearance. Finally, body image affect refers to the emotional experiences that derive from body-related evaluations.

9.2 Internal and External Body Image

A poor perception of mental body image can cause physical, mental, and psychological consequences. Sexual desire [4] and BI are correlated, so much so that physical appearance has been reported as a significant factor in women's sexual fantasies [5]. The evaluation of body image can influence interest in creating a sexual relationship, as well as the individual's sexual activity [6].

The study by Seal BN et al. [7], for example, examined the relationships among body self-esteem, sexual response to eroticism in a laboratory context, and self-reported sexual functioning in a nonclinical sample of 85 university women.

The women participated in a study session, during which mental sexual arousal, perceptions of physical arousal, and sexual desire were evaluated. The results showed that higher body self-esteem was significantly positively correlated with sexual desire in response. Similarly, higher body self-esteem was positively correlated with self-reported measures of sexual desire.

The subscales of sexual attractiveness and weight concern of the Body Esteem Scale, (which refer to body characteristics) were particularly linked to sexual desire. This is the first study to demonstrate that body self-esteem is correlated with sexual responses to a standardized erotic stimulus in a laboratory environment.

Having a positive body image accompanies a pleasurable sexual life and a constant desire. Feeling satisfied with the body and possessing a positive body image of oneself can lead to maximum self-esteem when creating a sexual relationship with one's partner [8]. Few international studies have dealt with the association between body image and sexual desire to reveal the negative impact of dissatisfaction and concern on women's sexual desire [9]. In particular, the study by Maserejian NN et al. [9] analyzed baseline data from 400 premenopausal patients with diagnosed HSDD. The function of sexual desire was measured using the *Female Sexual Function Index* (FSFI).

Over 85% of women reported multiple factors that contributed to the continued decrease in desire. The most commonly cited contributing factors were: "stress or fatigue" (60.0%), "dissatisfaction with my physical appearance" (40.8%), and inability to achieve orgasm (33.5%).

Exploratory analyses of the FSFI score confirmed that self-image and other sexual problems were significantly associated with decreased desire. Almost all participants (96%) were currently in a couple relationship. Antidepressant medications were currently used by 18.0% of women, hormonal contraceptives by 28.5%, and hormonal drugs by 7.3%. Physical functioning was consistent with the norms of the general population, while overall mental functioning was slightly lower.

Most of the scientific literature has revealed that the duration of a relationship, chronic diseases, negative body image, and body attractiveness are associated with HSDD [10]. These results imply an inverse association between marriage duration and sexual desire. In research on **356** women aged 20–70, it was found that women with marriage duration of 20–29 years had experienced higher levels of low sexual desire.

Specifically, the research of Murray SH et al. [11] *examined the duration of the relationship and its effect on sexual desire in a sample of 170 male and female university students aged between 18 and 25 years.*

The results indicated that women's sexual desire was significantly, negatively predicted by the duration of the relationship after controlling for age, relationship satisfaction, and sexual satisfaction. Men's sexual desire, however, was not significantly influenced by the duration of their romantic relationships.

These results suggest that men and women may have different experiences with sexual desire as relationships progress and that sexual desire may be influenced by different factors depending on gender.

In the study by Hoyt & Kogan et al. [12], it was highlighted that women dissatisfied with their sex lives reported greater body image dissatisfaction compared to those who felt satisfied. **On the other hand**, the research by Carvalho in Portugal et al. [13] showed that sexual desire is conditioned by relational passivity and the absence of erotic thoughts, but not by beliefs about body image.

In this particular study, 237 patients who responded to a series of questionnaires to *assess psychopathology, cognitive-emotional factors, dyadic adjustment, the presence of medical conditions, and menopause were evaluated.*

Psychopathology was measured by the Brief Symptom Inventory (BSI), and dysfunctional sexual beliefs by the Sexual Dysfunctional Beliefs Questionnaire, and thoughts and emotions in the sexual context by the Sexual Modes Questionnaire. Dyadic adjustment was assessed using the Dyadic Adjustment Scale. Medical condition was evaluated through the Medical History Formulation, and sexual desire was measured by the Sexual Desire subscale of the Female Sexual Function Index.

The results indicated that psychoticism was the only psychopathological dimension that significantly predicted sexual desire. Conservative beliefs and age-related beliefs were significant predictors of desire. Furthermore, the lack of erotic thoughts, thoughts of sexual failure and disengagement, as well as thoughts related to female passivity during sexual activity, *were significant predictors of desire*. Regarding relationship dimensions, dyadic cohesion and dyadic affection were the best predictors of sexual desire. Postmenopausal women and women with medical problems had reduced sexual desire. Lastly, thoughts of failure or disengagement during sexual activity were the only significant predictive factors of sexual desire in women with hypoactive sexual desire disorder (HSDD.)

9.2.1 HSDD in Pregnancy

One particular research on HSDD and pregnancy was conducted by Malary M et al. [14]. Data were collected using three tools: *a checklist of related factors, the Female Sexual Interest and Desire Inventory (SIDI-F), and the revised Female Sexual Distress Scale (FSD-R).* To assess body image satisfaction (BI), participants were asked to express their opinion *on how physically attractive they were before and during pregnancy using a 3-point Likert scale, ranging from not very attractive to very attractive* [15].

A total of **314** questionnaires were sent to four obstetric and gynecological centers, and 307 were returned. In total, 12 were excluded because they were incomplete [7] and based on exclusion criteria [5]. **The final sample consisted of 295 pregnant women aged between 18 and 40 years.**

Based on the SIDI-F cut-off score, 166 (56.3%) women were at risk of low sexual desire (29.2 ± 10.3). The average FSD-R score for this group (mean ± SD) was 5.55 ± 6.56, with 51 pregnant women (17.3%) scoring higher than the clinical cut-off score of 11. Among the 166 participants who were found to be at risk of low sexual desire by SIDI-F, 42 (25.3%) scored 11 or higher on FSD-R. *In other words, out of the 259 participants, 42 (14.2%) scored 33 or lower on SIDI-F and 11 or higher on FSD-R.*

Factors associated with a lower likelihood of low sexual desire were found to be satisfaction with foreplay, high dissatisfaction with sexual activity before and during pregnancy, increased frequency of intercourse in the previous month, and evolving body image. It should also be noted that the rate of sexual discomfort in this study was lower than those found in Canadian and American population-based studies of pregnant women: patients reported 40% sexual discomfort during pregnancy and unsatisfactory body image [16].

Moreover, the study by Lo SST et al. [17] highlighted that self-perception of low attractiveness was associated with both sexual problems and discomfort in young nonpregnant women. This research was conducted between November 2015 and June 2017, recruiting 431 young women who had turned to three clinics for sexual discomfort. The patients completed an anonymous questionnaire that detailed their demographic data, sexual behavior, current sexual relationship, sexual function, and sexual discomfort. *Sexual function and discomfort were assessed using the Female Sexual Function Index (FSFI) and the Female Sexual Distress Scale-Revised (FSDS-R).*

Overall, self-perception of one's body as unattractive to the boyfriend, not taking the initiative in intimacy, willingness for vaginal penetration, and absence of stress factors in life were associated with both sexual problems and discomfort.

The body image of pregnant women is an issue that should be further investigated by professionals in the field, especially considering that maternal and child health has gained such importance. The study by Meireles JF et al. [18] analyzed the literature on body image and body dissatisfaction among pregnant women. The research was based on articles extracted from the Scopus, PubMed, BVS, and PsycINFO databases, cross-referencing "pregnancy" with the keywords "body image" and "body dissatisfaction".

Once the inclusion and exclusion criteria were adopted, 40 studies were analyzed. These produced inconclusive data on body dissatisfaction during pregnancy. Symptoms of depression, low self-esteem, an inadequate approach to healthy eating, and weight gain beyond recommended limits were associated with a negative body image. The contradictory results could be related to the different tools used to measure body image.

9.3 Food, HSDD and Body Image in Adolescence

There is scientific evidence that an unhealthy body image (BI) is linked to obesity and physical inactivity, playing a key role in the onset of eating disorders—already during adolescence—and hypoactive desire. Our body image is a dynamic feature that can change over the course of life, but the stage of adolescence is crucial for the development of a healthy BI due to the age-related transitions that occur during this developmental period [19].

The influence of body ideals interacts with the critical period of adolescence, characterized by rapid, diversified physical changes that include changes in primary and secondary sexual characteristics, body shape, size, and composition. Key influences on body image include the media, which target adolescents, and peers, who contribute to perceived beliefs about the body ideal. In particular, the mass media can lead adolescents to internalize the ideals of physical attractiveness and beauty of Western society, leading to body dissatisfaction when these standards are perceived as unmet [20].

Recent findings have also shown that increased use of social media—such as Instagram and Snapchat—is associated with greater body dissatisfaction [21]. In line with sociocultural models of the development of body dissatisfaction and eating disorders [22], pressures on appearance from peers, family, and media, as well as psychological processes, contribute to the onset and persistence of body dissatisfaction and the consequent hypoactive sexual desire.

Many studies have particularly emphasized *body dissatisfaction in females*, due to their greater dissatisfaction and the prevailing desire to be thinner, with significant differences between real and ideal silhouettes [23]. ***The pattern in the two genders is indeed different, with higher female body dissatisfaction (BID), indicating the greater importance given by women to physical appearance compared to men***.

The relationship between body dissatisfaction and BMI was found to be linear in women [24]. In men, lesser dissatisfaction was observed, although this applies to both overweight individuals, who wish to be thinner, and underweight individuals, who wish to be more muscular. The relationship between body image dissatisfaction (BID) and BMI appears to be curvilinear [25].

Gualdi-Russo E. et al. [26] conducted a systematic review of articles published in the 10 years up to June 2022, according to the *PRISMA* statement, using the electronic databases *MEDLINE* and *Web of Science* (639 records) to summarize the literature on the relationship between body image dissatisfaction (BID) in adolescents (10–18 years), taking into account BMI and/or weight status.

All articles were independently reviewed using inclusion/exclusion criteria, data retrieved, and quality assessed with the Newcastle- *Ottawa* scale adapted for observational studies.

The main finding of interest from the majority of the 28 included studies is the negative association between body image dissatisfaction (BID) and physical activity (PA) during adolescence: as PA increases, BID decreases.

But there is more.

Various physical, cultural, social, and psychological changes that characterize early and middle adolescence interact with body image (BI) and BID between the ages of 10 and 18, as well as the resulting HSDD. Limiting to physical changes during this period, there are sex-specific differences that result in an increase in body fat mass and a decrease in lean mass in females compared to males, with consequent changes in body shape and size. However, a well-known decline in physical activity practice during adolescence [27] leads especially girls being less active than boys and not following WHO recommendations of at least 60 minutes of moderate to vigorous physical activity (MVPA) per day [28].

As confirmed by this research with a percentage of inactivity that is almost three times that of females compared to males in Spain [29] and exceeds 80% of inactivity in Brazilian girls [30] with less than 10% of girls participating in the recommended 60 min/day of MVPA for 7 days in the USA [31].

Inactivity in China was high (about 60%) but similar in both sexes [32] while in Indonesia girls met the daily physical activity recommendations slightly less than boys [33]. The only exception is the high averages of MVPA (over 5 hours per day, value not disaggregated by sex) reported for Ghanaian adolescents [34].

9.4 Do Doctors Suffer from HSDD and Unsatisfactory Body Image?

Since doctors are also human, Xing Tan et al. [35] investigated the relationship between HSDD, body image, and burnout among doctors.

The questionnaires used were Arizona sexual experience scale and the Chinese version of the Maslach burnout inventory–human service survey to assess sexual function and burnout among doctors in a primary hospital. Considering the doctors' work environment, the doctor-patient relationship, and sleep quality were also evaluated.

A total of 382 doctors were recruited; the prevalence of sexual dysfunction was 33.51%. HSDD and arousal disorders were the main sexual dysfunctions faced by male and female doctors, respectively. The prevalence of burnout among doctors was 43.72%.

The prevalence of sexual dysfunction among doctors who experienced burnout (45.51%) was higher than that observed in doctors without burnout (24.19%). Doctors with burnout showed significantly higher total and individual scores on the Arizona sexual experience scale compared to doctors without burnout (all P values <0.05). A significant positive correlation was found between inadequate body image and sexual desire, sexual arousal, lubrication, orgasm or erection, and sexual satisfaction. Further analysis confirmed that, in addition to burnout, dissatisfaction with one's physicality, income, a poor doctor-patient relationship, and poor sleep quality were significant factors contributing to HSDD among doctors in primary hospitals.

9.5 Conclusions

Body dissatisfaction plays an important role in general in HSDD. The study by Jones BA et al. [36] extended the investigation of HSDD into *gender dysphoria.* In some individuals, body dissatisfaction seems to manifest as eating disorders in order to suppress the body characteristics of the birth gender and to accentuate the characteristics of the gender identity. To date, no systematic review of the literature on body dissatisfaction and eating disorders in transgender individuals has been conducted. *This review found three studies that explored eating disorders in trans people, five studies that explored body image and eating disorders in trans people, and 18 studies that explored body image in trans people.*

The results of this review suggest that body dissatisfaction is fundamental to the discomfort experienced by transsexuals and that this dissatisfaction can also put some individuals at risk of developing eating disorders, as well as HSDD and psychiatric disorders. Furthermore, the results seem to suggest that the treatment of gender dysphoria is successful in improving and adapting to the evolving body image [36].

References

1. Abdo CH, Valadares AL, Oliveira WM Jr, Scanavino MT, Afif-Abdo J. Hypoactive sexual desire disorder in a population-based study of Brazilian women: associated factors classified according to their importance. Menopause. 2010;17:1114–21.
2. Muth JL, Cash TF. Attitudes towards body image: what difference does gender make? J Appl Soc Psychol. 1997;27:1438–52.
3. Cash TF, Fleming EC. The impact of body image experiences: development of the body image quality of life inventory. Int J Eat Disord. 2002;31:455–60.
4. Levine MP, Piran N. The role of body image in the prevention of eating disorders. Body Image. 2004;1:57–70.
5. McClintock EA. Handsome wants as handsome does: physical attractiveness and gender differences in revealed sexual preferences. Biodemography Soc Biol. 2011;57:221–57.
6. Cash TF, Maikkula CL, Yamamiya Y. "Baring the body in the bedroom": body image, sexual schemas and sexual functioning among college women and men. Electron J Hum Sex. 2004;7:1–9.
7. Seal BN, Bradford A, Meston CM. The association between body esteem and sexual desire among college women. Arch Sex Behav. 2009;38(5):866–72.
8. Woertman L, Van den Brink F. Body image and female sexual functioning and behavior: a review. J Sex Res. 2012;49:184–211.
9. Maserejian NN, Shifren JL, Parish SJ, Braunstein GD, Gerstenberger EP, Rosen RC. The presentation of hypoactive sexual desire disorder in premenopausal women. J Sex Med. 2010;7:3439.
10. Terimourpour N, Bidokhti NM, Pourshahbaz A. The relationship between attachment styles and sexual desire among Iranian women. Procedia Soc Behav Sci. 2011;30:108–12.

11. Murray SH, Milhausen RR. Sexual desire and relationship duration in young men and women. J Sex Marital Ther. 2012;38:28–40.
12. Hoyt WD, Kogan LR. Satisfaction with body image and peer relationships for males and females in a college environment. Sex Roles. 2001;45:199–215.
13. Carvalho J, Nobre P. Predictors of women's sexual desire: the role of psychopathology, cognitive-emotional determinants, relational dimensions, and medical factors. J Sex Med. 2010;7:928–37.
14. Malary M, Moosazadeh M, Keramat A, Sabetghadam S. Factors influencing low sexual desire and sexual distress in pregnancy: a cross-sectional study. Int J Reprod Biomed. 2021;19(10):909–20.
15. Kafy A, Alamoudi R, Alkafy S, Qary R. Female sexual function during pregnancy: a comparative cross-sectional study in Saudi Arabia. Glob J Res Anal. 2019;8:85–9.
16. Vannier SA, Rosen NO. Sexual discomfort and sexual problems during pregnancy: associations with sexual and relational satisfaction. J Sex Med. 2017;14:387–95.
17. Lo SST, Kok WM. Prevalence and risk factors for sexual problems and distress in young unmarried Chinese women: an observational study. J Sex Med. 2018;15:1620–8.
18. Meireles JF, Neves CM, de Carvalho PH, Ferreira ME. Body dissatisfaction among pregnant women: an integrative review of the literature. Ciênc Saúde Colet. 2015;20(7):2091–103.
19. Voelker DK, Reel JJ, Greenleaf C. Weight status and body image perceptions in adolescents: current perspectives. Adolesc Health Med Ther. 2015;6:49–58.
20. Gualdi-Russo E, Rinaldo N. Anthropometry and body image perception. In: Sineo L, Moggi CJ, editors. Manual of anthropology. Turin, Italy: UTET; 2022. p. 491–6.
21. Vuong AT, Jarman HK, Doley JR, McLean SA. Social media use and body dissatisfaction in adolescents: the moderating role of internalization of thinness and muscularity ideals. Int J Environ Res Public Health. 2021;18:13222.
22. Thompson JK, Heinberg LJ, Altabe M, Tantleff-Dunn S. Demanding beauty. In: Theory, assessment, and treatment of body image disorder. Washington, DC: American Psychological Association; 1999.
23. Gualdi-Russo E, Rinaldo N, Masotti S, Bramanti B, Zaccagni L. Sex differences in body image perception and ideals: analysis of possible determinants. Int J Environ Res Public Health. 2022;19:2745.
24. Kostanski M, Fisher A, Gullone E. Current conceptualization of body image dissatisfaction: have we got it wrong? J Child Psychol Psychiatry. 2004;45:1317–25.
25. Frederick DA, Peplau LA, Lever J. The swimsuit issue: correlations of body image in a sample of 52,677 heterosexual adults. Body Image. 2006;3:413–9.
26. Gualdi-Russo E, Rinaldo N, Zaccagni L. Physical activity and body image perception in adolescents: a systematic review. Int J Environ Res Public Health. 2022;19(20):13190.
27. Duarte LS, Palombo CNT, Solis-Cordero K, Kurihayashi AY, Steen M, Borges ALV, Fujimori E. The association between body weight dissatisfaction with unhealthy eating behaviors and lack of physical activity in adolescents: a systematic review. J Child Health Care. 2021;25:44–68.
28. Physical Activity (World Health Organization) [(accessed on 30 August 2022)]; available online: https://www.who.int/en/news-room/fact-sheets/detail/physical-activity
29. Fernández-Bustos JG, Infantes-Paniagua Á, Gonzalez-Martí I, Contreras-Jordán OR. Body dissatisfaction in adolescents: differences based on sex, BMI, and type and organization of physical activity. Int J Environ Res Public Health. 2019;27:3109.
30. Miranda VPN, Morais NS, Faria ER, Amorim PRDS, Marins JCB, Franceschini SDCC, Teixeira PC, Priore SE. Body dissatisfaction, physical activity and sedentary behavior in female adolescents. Rev Paulo Pediatr. 2018;36:482–90.
31. Robbins LB, Ling J, Resnicow K. Demographic differences and correlates of perceived discrepancy in body image among urban adolescent girls: a cross-sectional study. BMC Pediatr. 2017;17:201.

32. Song L, Zhang Y, Chen T, Maitusong P, Lian X. Association between body perception and food weight management behaviors among children and adolescents aged 6 to 17 years in China: cross-sectional study using CHNS (2015). BMC Public Health. 2022;22:175.
33. Niswah I, Rah JH, Roshita A. The association of body image perception with eating and physical activity behaviors among adolescents in Indonesia. Food Nutr Bull. 2021;42:S109–21.
34. Michels N, Amenyah SD. Body size ideals and dissatisfaction in Ghanaian adolescents: role of media, lifestyle and Well-being. Public Health. 2017;146:65–74.
35. Xing Tan Y, Tian T-TZ, Ge P-P, Wang Q-J, Chen R, Rong-Hui X, Meng X-J, Zhang T-T. Relationship between sexual dysfunction and burnout among doctors in primary hospital: a cross-sectional study. J Sex Med. 2024:qdae147.
36. Jones BA, Haycraft E, Murjan S, Arcelus J. Body dissatisfaction and disordered eating in trans people: a systematic review of the literature. Int Rev Psychiatry. 2016;28(1):81–94.

HSDD: National Differences in Doctor-Patient Communication

10

Abstract

Although it is crucial in establishing patient-centered care, doctor-patient communication is, in any context, a complex phenomenon. Its complexity increases when considering patients from different social backgrounds. Some studies have indicated that patients' experiences in healthcare vary among different sociodemographic groups. *The communication style of doctors tends to change based on the educational background of the patient: those with a lower level of education tend to be less informed, less involved in treatment decisions, are approached in a more directive and dominant manner, and are asked to take on greater responsibility for their own care* (Aelbrecht, Patient Educ Couns 102:776–81, 2019).

Keywords

Education · Ethnicity · Language barriers · Medical communication · Patient perspective · Health policy · Patient experience · Practice management · Quality improvement · Research studies · Doctor-patient communication guide

10.1 Introduction

It has been suggested that patient-centered communication does not necessarily translate into a **unique** approach, but rather that doctors should use a flexible, and **individualized** style for each patient. The study by Zandbelt LC et al. [2] examined the variability in patient-centered behavior in encounters with medical specialists and determined whether patient, visit, and doctor characteristics influence this variability. Thirty residents and specialists in internal medicine at a university hospital in the Netherlands, and 323 patients who had outpatient follow-up appointments (recorded via video), were recruited. Doctors and patients completed a questionnaire before the encounter.

E. V. Longhi, *Hypoactive Sexual Desire Disorder*,
https://doi.org/10.1007/978-3-032-00659-2_10

Consultations were coded using the **Patient-Centred Behavior Coding Instrument (PBCI)**. *The patient-centered behavior of doctors was determined by behaviors that facilitated, rather than inhibited, the patient's expression of their own perspective*. The results show that doctors differ in their communicative behavior: some have a more "patient-centered" communication style or show intra-individual variation, *adapting their style according to the individual circumstance*.

More often than not, doctors showed more facilitating behavior when patients were older, reported more physical symptoms, when they assessed the patients' health conditions as more severe, and when the doctor was a woman.

They showed more inhibitory behavior when patients reported more physical symptoms and when the doctor assessed the patients' health conditions as more severe. ***Apparently, sicker patients were targets of both greater facilitation and greater inhibition***. The variability in doctors' facilitating or inhibitory behavior was explained by patient characteristics, namely age and health conditions, and—except for the gender of the doctor— not by the characteristics of the doctor or the visit. This indicates that patient-centered doctor behavior is related to the type of patient being seen, especially regarding the severity of symptoms.

But when faced with a diagnosis of HSDD, the difficulties become glaring unless it is the patient who opens the discussion about their own sexuality, even when HSDD or sexual dysfunctions are the consequence of a chronic disease.

For this purpose, the study by Fuertes JN et al. [3], examined the cognitive and emotional characteristics of the doctor-patient relationship—*therapeutic alliance*—in relation to patients' beliefs about the usefulness of treatment (perceived utility), patients' beliefs about their ability to adhere to treatment (self-efficacy beliefs in adherence), patients' adherence to the treatment plan (adherence), and patient satisfaction.

Fifty-one men and 67 women, with an average age of 38.9 years, were recruited. Seventy-two were Euro-American, 23 African-American, 6 Asian-American, 11 Hispanic, and 6 of other nationalities. They reported an average of 7.3 years since the diagnosis of a chronic disease and an average of 7.1 doctor visits in the past year. *The patients' conditions included HIV/AIDS, hypertension, diabetes, asthma, and cancer*.

The results showed relationships from (moderate to strong) between therapeutic alliance and perceived utility, self-efficacy, adherence, and satisfaction. These premises also resulted not only in patient satisfaction but also in a more lasting therapeutic contract.

With patients increasingly seeking health information online [4], the Internet is playing a significant role in the distribution and amplification of often inaccurate scientific and therapeutic claims. False health information is estimated to constitute 11% of 2805 health-related websites [5].

Many scientific and medical institutions make significant efforts to inform patients about the potential harms associated with unproven interventions and therapies. The *Mayo Clinic* and other organizations have all supported patient education and public engagement in this area [6]. Despite such notable efforts, it is unclear whether these messages reach patients and whether patients consider these sources reliable and trustworthy [7].

10.2 How Do Doctors-Patients Communicate in Various Countries?

A study by *Donaldson CD* et al. [8] examined the differences in the quality of care ($N = 6945$), using the ***Hospital Consumer Assessment of Healthcare Providers and Systems*** (HCAHPS) survey. Data were collected between January 2014 and April 2019.

Bivariate and multivariate analyses evaluated the relationships between ethnicity and language with individual elements that capture specific components of care and overall hospital ratings, using regression modeling.

Compared to non-Hispanic white English-speaking patients, Hispanic/Latinx Spanish-speaking patients reported more positive interactions with nurses, doctors, the hospital environment, and a better understanding of care after discharge. The results also indicated that Hispanic/Latinx Spanish-speaking patients were more satisfied with their experience than non-Hispanic white patients.

Conversely, research by Rollins A et al. [9] investigated reports of Latinx populations reporting lower levels of patient-centered care and satisfaction in the United States, compared to their non-Latinx white counterparts. A literature review was conducted in *Ovid Medline*, *CINAHL*, and *PsycINFO*. Articles were excluded if they were not applicable to the healthcare sector, did not include a patient experience tool, or did not include Latinx or Spanish-speaking patients in the study population. Data extraction was performed for measured concepts, study dimensions, population, healthcare setting, and validated languages.

This review identified 224 manuscripts. Of these, 81 met the full inclusion criteria and represented 60 unique tools. These covered six categories: general patient experience (43%), experiences of discrimination and distrust (12%), cultural factors (10%), patient-provider relationship (10%), and communication (8%). Just over a third of the tools ($n = 24$, 5 pediatric, 19 adult) were validated in Spanish, and another 14 (23%) were validated only in English. Finally, 4 (7%) tools were identified that were developed for use in a language-concordant context.

Clinical research also suggests that patients and families from underrepresented minorities may experience lower rates of coordinated or patient-centered care, and these discrepancies can negatively impact care [10]. In another survey, parents interviewed in Spanish with an interpreter were three times more likely to be dissatisfied with their child's care.

They also reported more frequently that healthcare services were not easy to pursue [11]. In addition to language barriers, the experience of Latinx patients appears to be influenced by marginalization, discrimination, and the overlapping challenges related to immigration status and cultural factors [12]. Taking this into account, Latinx individuals report fundamentally different care experiences.

Furthermore, an accurate assessment of the patient experience not only contextualizes the unique cultural, social, and demographic factors among a vulnerable population, but also helps generate potential interventions to provide more patient-centered care [13].

10.3 Communication Questionnaires

In particular, the study by Donaldson CD et al. [8] used five tools that focused mainly on communication or health competence, all of which were validated in at least one language.

Three validated tools measure communication: the Perceived Efficacy in Patient-Physician Interactions (PEPPI), the Communication Assessment Tool (CAT), and the Parents Perception of Primary Care [14].

The PEPPI and CAT evaluated the ease of asking questions, explanations of the main concern, the ability to understand information, and listening skills. The *Parents Perception of Primary Care* also considers explanations of common content for primary care pediatric visits [15]. Two additional validated tools focused on health competence, including the Short Test of Functional Health Literacy in Adults (S-TOFHLA) and the Parent-Patient Activation Measure (P-PAM), both developed for use in Spanish-speaking patients [15]. The P-PAM focuses on a parent's confidence in their ability to understand their child's health problems, treatments, preventive health, and to communicate concerns to their doctor. The S-TOFHLA, on the other hand, uses a 7-minute reading comprehension test and a scoring system that assesses health literacy but no other domain.

Considering this, what would be the impact on a parent facing a child's sexual pathology? What kind of language would the specialist use if they feel unprepared to talk about sexuality in front of a minor? And if the same parent has difficulty addressing this topic because they are dysfunctional in intimacy?

There are six tools that primarily address with patient-healthcare provider relationships, evaluating three subdomains: decision-making process, trust, and empathy. Four validated tools deal with the decision-making process: the Shared Decision Making Q9 (SDM-Q9), CollaboRATE, Pediatric Family Satisfaction ICU-24, and the Lopez breast cancer survey [16].

The SDM-Q9 focuses on the patient's participation in planning and decision making, as well as satisfaction in evaluating treatment options.

CollaboRATE, a much shorter tool, primarily focuses on the patient's perception of a provider's effort to achieve these goals.

The ICU-24 survey also covers how much the patient and family felt included in the decision-making process while their child was in the intensive care unit (ICU), control over care, ease of understanding information, and specific ICU satisfaction domains.

The last tool, focused on the decision making process, the Lopez breast cancer survey, focused solely on breast surgery treatment, and suggestions [17].

Regarding discrimination and mistrust: the Experiences of Discrimination Scale (EOD), the Medical Mistrust Index (MMI), the Group-Based Medical Mistrust Scale (GBMMS), and the Perceived Ethnic Discrimination Questionnaire–Community Version (PEDQ-CV).

The EOD measured global level discrimination; including contexts, attitudes, and concern about experiences of discrimination; the PEDQ-CV in particular was validated in primary care contexts [18]. The GBMMS was developed for use in a medical context and measures mistrust in doctors, perception of care, and discrimination by healthcare providers [19]. The MMI was also developed for use in a medical context, but focuses on mistrust within the American healthcare system as a whole [20].

10.4 Further

The tools included the Tucker-Culturally Sensitive Health Care Inventory (T-CSHCI-PF), the CAHPS Cultural Competence Survey, and the Patient-Reported Clinician's Cultural Sensitivity Survey (PRCCS). Despite the plurality of investigative tools, the fact remains that linguistic, religious, political, and social differences significantly influence doctor-patient communication, especially in sexuality. An HSDD of an English-speaking patient differs from that of an Italian, Western in general or Asian culture. Thus, prejudices and habits of sexual relations between individuals greatly influence the feeling of discomfort or embarrassment in describing sexual dysfunctions and HSDD.

Ignoring these variables means making only abstract diagnoses and not individualized ones for the single patient, and the cultural, religious, social habits that belong to them.

A study by TIMMIS, C.L. et al. [21] investigated language barriers in healthcare for Latino populations in the United States through a systematic review of studies published in *Biomedical Journals* from 1990 to 2000. The aspects of the problem examined were access to healthcare, quality of care, and health status, health outcomes.

Five (55%) of the nine studies examining access to care found a significant negative effect of language; three (33%) found conflicting or weak evidence that language influenced access. Six (86%) of the seven studies evaluating the quality of care found a significant negative effect due to language barriers.

The evidence was conflicting regarding the level of importance attributable to language when considering access to care; however, non-English language status was an indicator of a population at risk of reduced access. Solid evidence showed that language barriers can negatively affect the quality of care.

10.5 Participation in Research Studies

The National Institutes of Health (NIH) is the world's largest public funder of research. In an attempt to make publicly funded data more accessible, NIH has established a new data management and sharing policy (DMS), effective from January 2023.

An interesting study [22] aimed to determine:

1. Participants' preferences on the types of data they are willing to share with external entities, and.
2. The participants' perspectives on the updated 2023 NIH data management and sharing policy.

A cross-sectional and nationally representative online survey was conducted among 610 English-speaking American adults in March 2023 using Prolific. Overall, 50% of the sample identified as female, 13% as Black or African American, and 7% as Hispanic or Latino, with an average age of 46 years. Most respondents (65%) agreed with the *National Institute Health* policy, but racial differences were noted with a higher percentage—28%—of Black participants indicating a decrease in willingness to participate in research studies with the updated policy in place. *Participants were more willing to share research data with healthcare providers*, but their preferences for data sharing varied depending on the type of data to be shared, and the recipients.

Participants were less willing to share sexual health and fertility data with health technology companies (41%) and public repositories (37%) compared to their healthcare providers (75%).

In response to the question about the new NIH data management and sharing policy, 302 (49%) participants provided written comments. The responses were divided: in support of the policy (33%), in favor of limiting data access (37%), prioritizing anonymity (17%), prioritizing autonomy (6%), and prioritizing transparency (22%).

Some participants supported the policy, appreciating its potential benefits, such as transparency and acceleration of research. However, many expressed concerns about the policy in ***relation to a loss of autonomy, fear of misuse of research data, lack of transparency, and lack of anonymity***. *Regarding concerns about loss of autonomy, participants felt they were the rightful custodians of their own data and should have control over the designation of data recipients, with one stating*: "**It is my information and I should be responsible for where it goes and who can access it**." (24-year-old woman). Other participants emphasized the importance of transparency in future uses of data, as one said, "**Although I agree that it can help make positive changes, I would 100% want to know which external companies they are talking about before being willing... it decreases my willingness [to participate]**." (54-year-old woman). Finally, many participants were aware of how difficult it is to truly anonymize data, which also raised significant concerns: "**By combining information from multiple sources, it is possible to de-anonymize**

data. "If you know my age, my zip code, and my income, you are very close to knowing who I am" (66-year-old man).

This shows that, while the NIH and research in human sciences move toward improving the accessibility of research data, it is crucial to maintain a balance that also safeguards patients' privacy and autonomy. While many participants expressed optimism about the 2023 NIH data management and sharing policy, individuals from underrepresented racial backgrounds expressed apprehension, which could be influenced by their knowledge of the history of unethical research studies and their experiences with current systemic inequalities in terms of access to healthcare and research today [23].

10.6 The Power of Communication

The relationship between communication and patient safety has underscored the importance of the relationship within the healthcare team, as well as specific training in doctor-patient communication for health care professionals [24].

Improved communication among healthcare teams has been associated with better quality patient care and greater patient satisfaction [25]. Conversely, communication failures have been found to be the most common cause of adverse events for patients and negative health outcomes.

At the University of Pittsburgh Medical Center [26], patient-doctor and patient-nurse communication were identified as areas of intervention to improve suboptimal patient satisfaction among inpatients in medicine.

In 2016, a total of **76** internal medicine residents and 85 medical service nurses participated. *The curriculum used teaching, video demonstrations, and role-playing, and was evaluated using pre-and post-surveys on participants' knowledge, attitudes, and confidence in health literacy*. Communication skills were evaluated using pre- and post-course direct observation with a communication skills checklist. ***The Hospital Consumer Assessment of Healthcare Providers and Systems (HCAHPS) scores were compared 3 months before and after the curriculum to assess changes in patient satisfaction***.

The communication skills of doctors were measured by comparing 205 pretraining and 168 posttraining patient consultations using a standardized checklist over a period of 6 months. The communication skills of nurses were measured by comparing 150 pretraining and 152 posttraining hospital discharges. Most skills significantly improved. If improving doctor-patient and nurse-patient communication is an important part of the therapeutic contract and patient satisfaction, we could advise the doctor to:

- Avoid rushing to make a diagnosis.
- Listen to the patient with empathy.
- Ask substantive and probing questions.

- Do not underestimate that HSDD has different characteristics from patient to patient, including relational factors, work concerns, mood disorders, food addictions, recent separation or divorce).
- Be patient in repeating the basic concepts of the diagnosis, using simple language—not necessarily medical.
- Prescribe essential clinical tests to exclude biological causes or pharmacological and surgical consequences.
- Positively note the wealth of information received from the patient, regardless of professional, cultural, religious level, and sexual habits.
- Pay attention to the partner in a stable relationship or to the characteristics usually chosen by the patient such as occasional partners.
- Avoid criticism and hasty judgments about previous consultations and what the patient reports about them.
- Consult the partner in a stable relationship when possible.
- Show humility in asking for the patient's patience in expanding the medical history to include the sexological evaluation (I need a sexological evaluation as well to offer you a more valid clinical plant).
- Any doubts the patient may have about the doctor's clinical hypotheses are due to their own anxiety and the disparity of information that the patient possesses, either summarized or obtained through the internet.
- Studies on doctor-patient communication emphasize that the therapeutic contract takes effect after 5 minutes of conversation.
- The introductory and farewell greetings with the patient can either instill superficiality or disinterest or, conversely empathy and agreement of intentions.
- The possible referral to the sexologist should not appear as a demand for responsibility but as an effort to build a team of specialists who will accompany the patient—without leaving him alone—in undertaking a therapeutic path, stages and outcome of which he is unaware.
- Patient satisfaction depends on the perception of not being treated as just one of many patients with HSDD but as an individual with particular factors for investigation and care.

10.7 Conclusions

A specific study by Irwin Goldstein et al. [27] examined the communication methods of doctors with patients suffering from hypoactive sexual desire disorder (HSDD), analyzing the language used by patients and doctors in the United States, France, and Germany when describing the symptoms, causes, and correlations of HSDD. A semi-structured interview was used, conducted independently and face-to-face with 127 doctors involved in the treatment of female sexual dysfunction (FSD), and 95 women with FSD screened for HSDD using a brief adaptation of the Sexual Interest and Desire Inventory–Female.

Doctors and patients found FSD to be a difficult topic to discuss. Recognition of the term HSDD was low, with a preference for "decreased sexual desire." Discomfort, currently an integral part of the diagnosis of HSDD, was an unpopular term. It implied for participants a state of fear or anxiety, as well as a degree of severity not reflected by their feelings about the condition. Key feelings conveyed by patients included low self-esteem, frustration, confusion, dissatisfaction or discontent, worry, anger, embarrassment, stress, depression, and a sense of incompleteness.

Doctors were frustrated by the lack of effective treatment options for HSDD, which contributed to reluctance in discussing sexual health with patients. Patients were increasingly motivated to seek treatment, with an "improvement in the level of desire" identified as the most significant treatment outcome, rather than an increase in satisfying sexual events.

More carefully constructed definitions, based on the understanding of common language between clinicians and patients, would improve doctor-patient communication and establish common expectations for the treatment of hypoactive sexual desire disorder. *Defining HSDD in simpler, nonpsychiatric terms such as "reduced sexual desire" illustrates how HSDD can be translated into more patient-friendly language.*

If that were not enough, the study by Harsh V, et al. [28] investigated the attitudes and practices of physicians regarding hypoactive sexual desire disorder (HSDD) in the context of primary care, using a self-administered questionnaire.

Fifty-three out of 155 physicians responded (46% response rate—41.5% women, 58.5% men). ***Of the respondents, 90% reported having little confidence in diagnosing HSDD***, 90% of physicians had not screened a patient for HSDD, and 98% of physicians had not prescribed medication to patients with HSDD. No significant gender differences were identified among physicians, but faculty members were more confident in diagnosing and treating HSDD compared to resident physicians.

The study by Gillen P. et al. [29] investigated how well physicians introduce themselves to patients, drawing inspiration from the "*hellomynameis*" campaign started by Dr. Kate Granger in the United Kingdom.

The survey was conducted over a period of 5 months by three qualified clinical observers on outpatient and inpatient patients.

A total of **353** patients were examined: 253 outpatients and 100 inpatients. One hundred and twenty-one were outpatients (47.8%), 73 were physicians (28.8%), while 59 (23.3%) were divided between obstetrics, gynecology, and ophthalmology. One hundred acute presentations were examined: 52% in the emergency department, 20% in the acute medical assessment unit, 21% in the acute surgical assessment unit, and 7% in other specialties or departments.

According to the returned forms, ***79% of doctors (n = 279) introduced themselves to patients. Eleven percent (39) of doctors did not introduce themselves, and 8.5% of patients (30) were unsure whether the doctor had introduced themselves***. Five patients left their responses blank. Consultants were significantly more likely (P = 0.02) to introduce themselves or shake hands compared to non-consultant hospital doctors. *Gender had no impact (P = 0.43) on introductions or handshakes, regardless of the doctor's rank.* Three hundred seventeen patients (89.7%) felt that an introduction made a positive difference in their healthcare visit. Thirty patients (8.5%) felt it made no difference, and eight patients (2.2%) were unsure or did not respond. Definitive evidence of an introduction was documented in 79% of patients with 14.5% not receiving or unable to recall whether an introduction was made during repeated visits. 6.5% reported not receiving any introduction. On this basis, *what kind of reflection might andrological or gynecological patients seeking a consultation for HSDD and for all sexual functions make? These are very delicate topics and difficult to disclose for all patients, conditioned by anxiety and feelings of inadequacy?*

It seems that the problem of doctor-patient communication is even global. Evidence of this is the study by Hayek S et al. [30] which investigated patient satisfaction in relation to the performance of primary care physicians (PCPs) and potential differences based on ethnicity in a multicultural population.

A national, cross-sectional telephone survey was conducted on a random sample of the Israeli population aged ≥25 years. The level of satisfaction derived from the performance of the PCP was evaluated using a validated questionnaire (30 items; 6 different domains).

The final sample included (n = 827 Jews; n = 605 Arabs, average age 54.7 (±14.9). Arab patients reported lower overall satisfaction with the performance of PCPs compared to Jews. Arabs reported lower satisfaction with the performance of PCPs in the following domains: communication skills; interpersonal manners and time spent with patients.

In terms of sexuality and HSDD, how much can these experiences influence the construction of a therapeutic contract?

References

1. Aelbrecht K, Hanssens L, Detollenaere J, Willems S, Deveugele M, Pype P. Determinants of physician–patient communication: the role of language, education and ethnicity. Patient Educ Couns. 2019;102(4):776–81.
2. Zandbelt LC, Smets EM, Oort FJ, Godfried MH, de Haes HC. Determinants of physicians' patient-centered behavior in the medical specialist encounter. Soc Sci Med. 2006;63(4):899–910. https://doi.org/10.1016/j.socscimed.2006.01.024. Epub 2006 Mar 13
3. Fuertes JN, Mislowack A, Bennett J, Paul L, Gilbert TC, Fontan G, Boylan LS. The physician-patient working alliance. Patient Educ Couns. 2007;66(1):29–36. https://doi.org/10.1016/j.pec.2006.09.013. Epub 2006 Dec 22
4. UnitedHealthcare. Executive summary of the UnitedHealthcare consumer sentiment survey; 2019, pp. 1–17.
5. Gregory J. Health websites are notoriously misleading. So we rated their reliability; 2019. www.statnews.com/2019/07/26/health-websites-are-notoriously-misleading-so-we-rated-their-reliability/
6. United States Food and Drug Administration. Statement on the permanent injunction of the stem cell clinic and the FDA's ongoing efforts to protect patients from the risks of unapproved products; 2019. www.fda.gov/news-events/press-announcements/statement-stem-cell-clinic-permanent-injunction-and-fdas-ongoing-efforts-protect-patients-risks
7. Master Z, Robertson K, Frederick D, Rachul C, Caulfield T. Stem cell tourism and public education: the missing elements. Cell Stem Cell. 2014;15(3):267–70.
8. Donaldson CD, Bharadwaj A, Giafaglione B, Patton P, Fortier MA, Kain ZN. Ethnicity and language differences in patient experience: an analysis of the HCAHPS survey. J Racial Ethn

Health Disparities. 2022;9(3):899–908. https://doi.org/10.1007/s40615-021-01029-0. Epub 2021 Mar 26

9. Rollins A, Wandell G, Epstein S, Bonilla-Velez J. Evaluating patient and family experience among Spanish-speaking and LatinX patients: a scoping review of existing instruments. J Racial Ethn Health Disparities. 2023;10(4):1878–98. https://doi.org/10.1007/s40615-022-01371-x. Epub 2022 Aug 1
10. Roncoroni J, Frank M, Hudson A, et al. Latin patients' perceptions of culturally sensitive healthcare and their association with patient satisfaction, patient-healthcare provider communication, and therapeutic alliance. J Racial Ethn Health Disparities. 2022;9(2):620–9.
11. Hsueh L, Hirsh AT, Maupomé G, Stewart JC. Patient-healthcare provider language concordance and health outcomes: a systematic review, evidence map, and research agenda. Med Care Res Rev. 2021;78(1):3–23.
12. Curt AM, Kanak MM, Fleegler EW, Stewart AM. Increasing inclusivity in patient-centered research begins with language. Prev Med (Baltim). 2021:149. https://doi.org/10.1016/J.YPMED.2021.106621.
13. Shirley E, Josephson G, Sanders J. Fundamentals of patient satisfaction measurement. Physician Leadersh J. 2016;3(1):12–7.
14. Krugman SD, Racine A, Dabrow S, et al. Measuring primary care for children in pediatric resident continuity practices: a continuity research network study. Pediatrics. 2007;120(2) https://doi.org/10.1542/peds.2006-1346.
15. DeCamp LR, Leifheit K, Shah H, et al. Cross-cultural validation of the parent-patient activation measure in low-income Spanish and English speaking parents. Patient Educ Couns. 2016;99(12):2055–62. https://doi.org/10.1016/j.pec.2016.07.003.
16. De las Cuevas C, Perestelo-Perez L, Rivero-Santana A, Cebolla-Martí A, Scholl I, Härter M. Validation of the Spanish version of the 9-item shared decision-making questionnaire. Health Expect. 2015;18(6):2143–53. https://doi.org/10.1111/hex.12183.
17. López ME, Kaplan CP, Nápoles AM, Hwang ES, Livaudais JC, Karliner LS. Satisfaction with the decision-making process and regret for the treatment among Latinas and non-Latina white women with DCIS. Patient Educ Couns. 2014;94(1):83–9. https://doi.org/10.1016/j.pec.2013.09.005.
18. Brondolo E, Kelly KP, Coakley V, et al. The questionnaire on perceived ethnic discrimination: development and preliminary validation of a community version. J Appl Soc Psychol. 2005;35(2):335–65. https://doi.org/10.1111/j.1559-1816.2005.tb02124.x.
19. Thompson HS, Valdimarsdottir HB, Winkel G, Jandorf L, Redd W. The group-based medical mistrust scale: psychometric properties and association with breast cancer screening. Prev Med (Baltim). 2004;38(2):209–18. https://doi.org/10.1016/j.ypmed.2003.09.041.
20. Sheppard VB, Huei-Yu Wang J, Hurtado-de-Mendoza A, Sutton AL, LaVeist TA. Psychometric properties of the medical mistrust index (MMI) in Latin immigrants. Behav Med. 2019;45(2):128–33. https://doi.org/10.1080/08964289.2019.1585326.
21. Timmins CL. The impact of language barriers on the health care of Latinos in the United States: a review of the literature and guidelines for practice. J Midwifery Womens Health. 2002;47(2):80–96. https://doi.org/10.1016/s1526-9523(02)00218-0.
22. Niño de Rivera S, Masterson Creber R, Zhao Y, Eslami S, Mangal S, Dugdale LS, Reading TM. Public perspectives on increased data sharing in health research in the context of the 2023 National Institutes of Health Data Sharing Policy. PLoS One. 2024;19(8):e0309161. https://doi.org/10.1371/journal.pone.0309161.
23. Scharff DP, Mathews KJ, Jackson P, Hoffsuemmer J, Martin E, Edwards D. More than Tuskegee: understanding mistrust in research participation. J Health Care Poor Underserved. 2010;21:879–97. https://doi.org/10.1353/hpu.0.0323.
24. Nelson S, White CF, Hodges BD, Tassone M. Training of interprofessional teams at the pre-license level: a review of the literature. Acad Med. 2017;92(5):709–16.
25. Townsend-Gervis M, Cornell P, Vardaman JM. Interdisciplinary rounds and structured communication reduce rehospitalizations and improve some outcomes for patients. West J Nurs Res. 2014;36(7):917–28.

26. Allenbaugh J, Corbelli J, Rack L, Rubio D, Spagnoletti C. A brief communication curriculum improves communication skills of residents and nurses and patient satisfaction. J Gen Intern Med. 2019;34(7):1167–73.
27. Goldstein I, Lines C, Pyke R, Scheld JS. National differences in patient-clinician communication regarding hypoactive sexual desire disorder. J Sex Med. 2009;6(5):1349–57. https://doi.org/10.1111/j.1743-6109.2008.01204.x.
28. Harsh V, McGarvey EL, Clayton AH. Physician attitudes regarding hypoactive sexual desire disorder in a primary care clinic: a pilot study. J Sex Med. 2008;5(3):640–5.
29. Gillen P, Sharifuddin SF, O'Sullivan M, Gordon A, Doherty EM. How good are doctors at introducing themselves? #hellomynameis. Postgrad Med J. 2018;94(1110):204–6. https://doi.org/10.1136/postgradmedj-2017-135402. Epub 2018 Jan 13
30. Hayek S, Derhy S, Smith ML, Towne SD Jr, Zelber-Sagi S. Patient satisfaction with primary care physician performance in a multicultural population. Isr J Health Policy Res. 2020;9(1):13.

HSDD and Sexual Violence in Patients with Arousal Difficulties

11

Abstract

Childhood traumatic events are known as developmental factors for various sexual and psychiatric disorders. One study (Tekin et al., Nord J Psychiatry. 70(2):88–92; 2016) analyzed data obtained from 113 patients with SAD. Childhood traumatic experiences were assessed using the ***Childhood Trauma Questionnaire and the Arizona Sexual Experience Scale***. Data from interviews conducted with Structured *Clinical Interview for DSM–IV Axis I Disorders* (SCID–I) were used for diagnosis determination. Each patient was administered the ***Beck Anxiety Scale, the Beck Depression Scale, and the Liebowitz Social Anxiety Scale***. A history of childhood physical abuse (CPA) was present in 45.1% of patients with SAD and HSDD: 14.2% had a history of childhood sexual abuse (CSA). A co-diagnosis of depression was present in 30.1% of patients with SAD and 36.3% had HSDD. The history of CSA and the co-diagnosis of depression were determined to be two strong predictors in patients with SAD.

Keywords

Childhood trauma · Depression · Sexual dysfunction · Social anxiety disorder, desire disorder and sexual dysfunctions, anxiety · Anxiety sensitivity · Depression · Emotion regulation · Sexual functioning

11.1 Introduction

Studies investigating childhood trauma in generalized anxiety disorder (SAD) suggest that parental emotional abuse towards the child (cursing, insults, denigration, and nonphysical aggression) and emotional neglect (emotional deprivation or the absence of feeling special, loved, or part of a protective environment) can be important factors in the development of SAD and hypoactive desire disorder.

E. V. Longhi, *Hypoactive Sexual Desire Disorder*,
https://doi.org/10.1007/978-3-032-00659-2_11

A Case—Raffaele, 61-year-old, an entrepreneur, exhibits hypoactive sexual desire disorder (HSDD) and anxiety-depressive disorder. Childhood ended for the patient at age 8. At the first sign of puberty, his mother reflexively said, "*Well, now you're an adult, go to work*." Raffaele describes years of working during the day, even in markets, and studying at night: he graduated at age 20 and earned an engineering degree at 55 without his mother's knowledge. Married, he met his wife at age 18, and his in-laws became his second family. He confided to his partner that, at age 9, he was abused by his best friend's older brother. Threatened by him not to tell anyone, the guilt and fear that this boy might report him to friends led him to refuse to speak for 2 years. His parents did not notice the mood change—"*I was a joyful and outgoing boy before then*." His mother labeled him as introverted. With his wife, sexuality is infrequent (she takes the initiative), and his lack of virility is a cause of reproach from her. They have no children, and the depression is underestimated by everyone, as is the HSDD. Why doesn't he confide? "*I feel like my own caregiver. If I asked my wife for help, I fear she would leave or scold me...* ".

Like many stories, studies on adults with social anxiety disorder (SAD) and disorder (HSDD) also indicate that these individuals report childhood experiences associated with emotional abuse and/or neglect. Individuals with SAD are more likely than controls to perceive that their parents used shame as a form of discipline [2].

Two separate studies [3] found that, compared to healthy non-anxious patients, patients with SAD described their parents as rejecting and lacking emotional warmth. In another study [4] it was found that parental rejection was associated with social anxiety.

Simon and colleagues [5] recently reported that *56% of individuals with SAD reported a history of childhood emotional abuse and 39% of individuals with SAD reported a history of childhood emotional neglect.* **Furthermore**, they recently examined the relationship between various types of childhood trauma and the severity of social anxiety, overall symptom severity, disability, resilience, and quality of life in a sample of adults with SAD and HSDD. A history of childhood emotional abuse or neglect was associated with greater severity of SAD and overall symptoms; emotional neglect was also associated with lower resilience. *Childhood sexual abuse was associated with greater disability, while physical abuse and childhood neglect were not associated with any of these psychological outcomes.*

11.2 Clinical Studies

In the study by Kuo JR et al. [6], a total of 102 patients, including 52 women, were recruited and administered the short form of the *Childhood Trauma Questionnaire* (CTQ-SF), a 28-item questionnaire compromising 25 clinical items and three validity items that assess **five specific forms of childhood trauma: sexual abuse** ("Someone tried to touch me in a sexual way or tried to make me touch them"), **physical abuse** ("I was punished with a belt"), physical neglect ("I had to wear dirty clothes"), **emotional abuse** ("People in my family called me 'stupid,' 'lazy,' or 'ugly'), and **emotional neglect** ("I felt unloved").

Respondents were asked to choose responses on a five-point Likert scale, ranging from *never to very often* [7].

Participants also completed questionnaires to assess clinical symptoms across different domains. The severity of social anxiety was measured using the *Social Interaction Anxiety Scale* (SIAS) [8], a 20-item self-report measure that assesses anxiety related to social interactions in dyads and groups. Additionally, the *State-Trait Anxiety Inventory* (STAI-T) [9], a well-established measure of trait anxiety with high test-retest reliability ($r = 0.73–0.86$), was used.

Depressive symptoms were measured using the *Beck Depression Inventory-II* (BDI-II) [10], a 21-item self-report measure of depressive symptoms assessed over the previous week.

To examine group differences in childhood trauma rates [11], the following parameters were considered: *sexual abuse ≥8, physical abuse ≥8, physical neglect ≥8, emotional abuse ≥10, emotional neglect ≥15*. The Mann-Whitney test [11] was then used to examine differences between groups in childhood trauma rates and in each trauma subtype.

11.3 Results

Individuals with social anxiety disorder (SAD) and hypoactive sexual desire disorder (HSDD) have higher levels of childhood emotional abuse and emotional neglect compared to the healthy control group (HC). There are no differences between groups in levels of childhood sexual abuse, physical abuse, or physical neglect.

In individuals with SAD and HSDD, childhood emotional abuse and neglect are associated with the severity of social anxiety in adulthood, generalized anxiety, depression, and self-esteem.

Patients with *Borderline Personality Disorder* (BPD) also exhibit altered sexual behavior, such as sexual avoidance or sexual impulsivity, which has been repeatedly linked to sexual trauma occurring in a high percentage of BPD patients. The study by *Schulte-Herbrüggen O* et al. [12], investigated sexual function and the impact of sexual trauma in female patients with BPD compared to a healthy control group.

Sexual function was measured using the *Female Sexual Function Index.* Additionally, diagnoses were made using the *Structured Clinical Interview for DSM-IV Axis II Disorders* (SCID-II) and the *Mini International Neuropsychiatric Interview* (MINI) for Axis I disorders. Sexual function was measured using the *Female Sexual Function Index* and the *Post-Traumatic Stress Disorder Scale* for trauma assessment. Sexual orientation was evaluated through self-assessment.

Forty-five women with borderline personality disorder (BPD), diagnosed according to DSM-IV criteria, and 30 healthy women completed questionnaires on sexual function and history of sexual abuse, as well as interviews on Axis I and II disorders and psychotropic medications. The BPD group showed a significantly higher prevalence of sexual dysfunction. Subgroup analyses revealed that BPD with concomitant sexual trauma, rather than BPD alone, better explains impaired sexual function. *Sexual inactivity was primarily related to current major depression or the use of selective serotonin reuptake inhibitors (SSRI) medications*. In sexually active participants, medications and depression symptoms did not significantly impact sexual function.

Furthermore, reviewing the scientific literature highlights that childhood sexual trauma can be considered a nonspecific risk factor for bipolar disorder. Additionally, *individuals with bipolar disorder also exhibit sexual identity disturbances and higher rates of homosexual relationships compared to non-bipolar disorder individuals*. Patients with bipolar disorder also BPD also exhibit greater sexual impulsivity compared to non-BPD individuals. Risky sexual behaviors among individuals with bipolar disorder are associated with higher rates of sexually transmitted diseases, unwanted pregnancies, rape, and commercial sexual relationships, especially among drug addicts. Although psychotherapy is widely recommended for bipolar disorder, few systematic studies have been conducted on the effect of these treatments on comorbid post-traumatic symptoms related to childhood sexual trauma.

11.4 Sexual Abuse and Body Image

Body shame in men and women has been associated with increased sexual self-consciousness, reduced sexual pleasure, and more sexual problems [13]. Research has shown that negative body evaluations during sexual activity can affect sexual functioning due to cognitive and affective interference and are significantly correlated with fewer sexual experiences, lower sexual assertiveness, increased anxiety, and sexual avoidance, [14] as well as hypoactive sexual desire disorder. Pujols et al. [15] found that various aspects of body image, including weight concern, physical condition, sexual attractiveness, and thoughts about a body (due to the abuse suffered) during sexual activity predict sexual satisfaction or repulsion in patients.

Sexual traumatization, such as childhood sexual abuse (CSA), appears particularly relevant to a person's attitudes towards their own body [16]. *This may be due to body areas that trigger potentially traumatic memories of the violation of one's physicality*. It has been found that body esteem related to sexual attractiveness is significantly lower in women and men with a history of CSA compared to nonabused individuals [17]. In one study, women who experienced sexual trauma demonstrated significantly more negative body evaluations compared to patients with nonsexual trauma or without a history of abuse.

Patients with histories of CSA [18] often develop sexual self-perceptions that integrate their early abuse, which can influence their adult sexuality. Women with a history of CSA reported conflicting tendencies towards seeking or avoiding sexual experiences, with both hypersexual and hyposexual tendencies [19]. Women with a history of CSA develop adaptive sexual responses after their abuse that may be influenced by their body evaluations and sexual self-perceptions [20].

The study by Finkelhor and Browne et al. [18] *also proposed that women often internalize blame and guilt for their early sexual abuse, which affects their adult sexuality by creating a fear or aversion to sexuality.* Previous research has shown that some patients with CSA histories exhibited increased **cortisol** [21] in response to sexual stimuli. *An increase in cortisol could represent a stress reaction to stimuli, which, in turn, could lead to inhibitory sexual responses*. The dual control model postulates perceptions of sexual stimuli as threatening, which would adaptively increase inhibition to avoid the threat [22].

Negative body perceptions of patients could play a role in dissociation during sexual activity, [14] ***such that women dissociate to avoid negative responses to their body, resulting in lower arousal responses***.

A history of childhood sexual abuse is a predictor of the risk of eating disorders and sexual dysfunction, [23] and has been repeatedly implicated in the development of a distorted body image and negative body evaluations in the eating disorder literature. Specifically, a history of childhood sexual abuse has been linked to the psychological dysregulation of behavioral activation, such as binge eating, and restriction, such as starvation, pathways [24] involved in eating disorders. The conceptual model of behavioral activation and restriction pathways implicated in eating disorders is similar to the arousal and inhibition pathways of the sexual response model of dual control [25].

Patients seeking medical consultation for sexual difficulties often present with additional personal or relational disorders and symptoms. This is particularly true when they have experienced cumulative adverse childhood experiences (CACE), which are associated with symptom complexity. ***CACE refers to the extent to which an individual has experienced an accumulation of different types of adverse childhood experiences, including sexual, physical, and psychological abuse; neglect; exposure to interparental violence; and bullying***.

The study by BRIGAS N et al. [26] recruited **307 patients**—men and women–aged 18 and over who sought consultation for sexual difficulties. They were administered: *Global Measure of Sexual Satisfaction Scale, Dyadic Adjustment Scale-4, Experiences in Close Relationships-12, Beck Depression Inventory-13, Trauma Symptom Inventory-2, and Psychiatric Symptom Inventory-14.*

The results showed that ***58.1% of women and 51.9% of men reported at least four forms of childhood adversity***. The average number of (ACEs) was 4.10 (SD = 2.23) in women and 3.71 (SD = 2.08) in men. Structural equation modeling showed that ACEs contribute directly and indirectly to sexual satisfaction in adults seeking sexual therapy through clinically significant individual and relational symptom complexities.

The results underscore the importance of addressing clinically significant psychological and relational symptoms that may arise from ACEs when treating sexual difficulties in adults seeking sexual therapy [27].

11.5 Partners of Abused Patients

The study by Rosen NO et al. [28] examined the sexual, relational, and emotional consequences for partners of patients with a history of abuse. Ninety-seven couples, where the partner suffered from *HSDD* and sexual disorders, and 108 control couples were recruited: they independently completed questionnaires related to sexual desire, sexual distress, sexual function, sexual satisfaction, sexual communication, relational satisfaction, depression, and anxiety.

In summary: *Sexual Desire Inventory-2; Female Sexual Distress Scale; Female Sexual Functioning Index; International Index of Erectile Functioning (IIEF), Global Measure of Sexual Satisfaction, Dyadic Sexual Communication Scale, Couple Satisfaction Index, Beck Depression Inventory-II, State-Trait Anxiety Inventory-Short Form.*

It emerged that partners of women with HSDD and sexual disorders reported *lower sexual satisfaction, poorer sexual communication, and greater sexual distress, compared to partners in the control group. Additionally, they reported more difficulties with orgasmic and erectile functioning and lower overall satisfaction and sexual relationship satisfaction on the International Index of Erectile Function (IIEF), compared to control partners.* Women with HSDD and sexual disorders reported hypoactive or absent desire and minimal or no sexual satisfaction, along with depressive and anxious symptoms, compared to both control group women and their own partners. Communication with the partner on sexual topics was entirely absent. *Women with HSDD and sexual disorders also reported lower sexual desire, arousal, lubrication, and satisfaction, and greater pain during intercourse on the Female Sexual Function Index compared to control group women.*

Women in a stable relationship with a partner are nearly 5 times more likely to be distressed by low desire and receive a diagnosis of HSDD and sexual disorder compared to women without a partner, indicating that interpersonal factors are highly relevant, although largely overlooked in past research [29].

Rosen NO et al. [29] **conducted** a cross-sectional, longitudinal, dyadic, study examining partner responses on the sexual, relational, and psychological well-being of couples and whether the effects persisted after 1 year. Eighty-nine patients diagnosed with hypoactive sexual desire disorder and sexual disorders were recruited; their partners reported on sexual desire, sexual satisfaction, relationship satisfaction, sexual distress, and anxiety. ***One year later, 66 couples completed the questionnaires again***: *Sexual Desire Inventory-Solitary and Partner-Focused, Global Measure of Sexual Satisfaction, Female Sexual Distress Scale, Couple Satisfaction Index, and State-Trait Anxiety Inventory-Short Form.*

When women with hypoactive sexual desire disorder and sexual disorders perceived more positive (supportive, compassionate) responses from their partners compared to negative (hostile, indifferent) responses, they were more satisfied with the relationship, and both they and their partners reported lower anxiety. When partners reported more positive than negative responses, they experienced greater sexual and relational satisfaction and less sexual distress and anxiety. Exploratory analyses revealed that the women's perceptions of their partners' responses explained the link between partner responses and the women's relationship satisfaction and anxiety. ***Partner responses did not predict any change in outcomes over time***.

11.6 Abuse, Urinary Symptoms and Related Conditions

Attempted or completed sexual abuse (SA) conducted without the victim's consent can involve penetrative [30] or non-penetrative and non-contact acts. The perpetrator of the abuse may be a complete stranger or someone familiar to the victim, and the acts can be committed in private or public spaces [31]. ***The prevalence of SA is widely underestimated; results from a recent survey suggest that 1 in 5 women and 1 in 59 men have been exposed to an attempted or completed rape in their lifetime***. Rates of childhood sexual abuse (CSA) can vary: between 2% and 62% of women and between 3% and 16% of men [32]. The reasons for underreporting by victims are multiple and may include feelings of shame, fear, and guilt; a risk of retaliation by the perpetrator; and [33] a lack of awareness that forced sexual acts constitute SA [34].

Abuse can have a profound impact on victims, ranging from reduced levels of global functioning to prolonged trauma-related symptoms and an increased risk of developing substance abuse.

Both male and female victims may report increased rates of depression, anxiety, suicidal ideation, post-traumatic stress disorder (PTSD), hypoactive sexual desire disorder (HSDD), dysfunctional urinary symptoms [35]. Multiple physical and psychological sequelae have been reported, including anxiety, anger, depression, re-victimization, self-harm, sexual difficulties, substance abuse, suicidal tendencies, impaired self-esteem, interpersonal problems, obsessions and compulsions, dissociation, and post-traumatic stress responses to somatization characterized by medically unexplained symptoms.

Urological symptoms are likely common among SA survivors. *A Dutch study suggested that 2.1% of men and 13% of women seeking urological care may report SA* [36].

Many of the physical and psychological sequelae of childhood sexual abuse persist into adulthood [37], and up to one-third of patients attending a gynecological clinic have experienced childhood sexual abuse [38]. Childhood sexual abuse victims under the age of 6 have more commonly reported urinary tract infections, daytime incontinence, and nocturnal enuresis [39].

Sexual abuse (SA) is likely underreported, and in the Dutch study, only 15% of participants with a history of SA had disclosed it to their urologist. In a study conducted in five Nordic countries, the majority of women did not disclose a history of SA to their gynecologist [40]. Seventy percent of Dutch urologists inquired about SA when taking the medical history [41]; however, the rates of inquiries may vary depending on medical specializations and different healthcare settings.

The cause of urinary incontinence was unclear, and the inclusion of validated questionnaires, and possibly urodynamics, in future studies would help determine whether incontinence was due to overactive bladder, stress incontinence, or a mixed condition. Micturition difficulties were reported less frequently, and the reported symptoms included pain during urination, hesitation, slow flow, dribbling, holding urine until it became painful, incomplete bladder emptying, weak urinary flow, and straining to initiate urination [42]. Questionnaires like the UDI-6 specifically investigate micturition difficulties; however, only the total score was reported in studies. Urinary retention was not reported, and post-void residual volumes were not measured in any of the studies; therefore, it was not possible to assess the extent of incomplete bladder emptying.

The age at which SA occurs is also significant; it has been shown that SA occurring during critical developmental periods causes profound endocrinological and immunological consequences that can have long-term effects on an individual's ability to react and respond to illness [43]. Somatic problems such as musculoskeletal pain, ear, nose, and throat symptoms, abdominal pain, and gastrointestinal symptoms, fatigue, and dizziness are more common in adults with a history of childhood trauma compared to non-traumatized counterparts. ***These subjective physical health problems, medically unexplained, often persist and present as functional somatic syndromes such as fibromyalgia, chronic fatigue, and irritable bowel syndrome*** [44], in addition to sexual dysfunctions and HSDD.

However, it is likely that there are different mechanisms responsible for LUTS in SA survivors. Physical trauma to the perineum and pelvis [45] can cause damage to regional anatomy. Some studies have demonstrated an association between LUTS and anxiety, depression [46], and PTSD [47]. The neurobiological mechanisms involve the corticotropin-releasing factor, as well as serotonergic and dopaminergic systems in the pathogenesis of mood disorders and PTSD, and possible links with LUTS. *There is a possibility that adverse life events may lead to neurobiological and physiological changes that increase the risk of both mood disorders and somatic disorders, but the risk factors may differ* [48]. Somatization may be an adaptive response to psychological distress [49], and although specific symptoms related to SA have not been consistently identified [50], it is plausible that LUTS may be associated with complex PTSD and served as a manifestation of somatization related to SA.

Pharmacologically, duloxetine, a serotonin and norepinephrine reuptake inhibitor (SNRI), which is well-established in the treatment of depression and anxiety, has been used with successfully in managing both overactive bladder (OAB) and stress urinary incontinence (SUI) [51].

11.7 Parents' Reaction

The study by Marriage ND et al. [51] evaluated parents' *ability to identify normal, concerning, and harmful sexualized behaviors in children and adolescents, as well as their ability to identify and select an appropriate level of intervention.*

The influence of a parent's relationship with the victim or perpetrator on the level of action taken was also examined. ***A cross-sectional survey determined that***

parents (N = 244) were unable to consistently and accurately identify sexualized behaviors and provided levels of intervention responses below those recommended.

Parents were more capable of identifying and responding to behaviors considered normal and age-appropriate but had greater difficulty with behaviors considered concerning or harmful.

They were significantly less able to accurately identify and respond to behaviors exhibited by very young children (in the age range of 0–4 years).

Since the lack of accurate knowledge of the risks and indicators of child sexual abuse negatively affects the ability to prevent and detect abuse, the findings have implications for a shift from a forensic model of child protection to a public health model, emphasizing parent and community education.

More in-depth, the study by COLE PM et al. [52] examined the educational attitudes of survivors of incestuous and non-incestuous child sexual abuse, as well as their perceptions of their parents' behavior. ***Forty*** *women with children completed questionnaires designed to assess their own educational behavior and that of their parents, in terms of dimensions of acceptance and parental control.*

The data indicated that women from incestuous backgrounds had more negative perceptions of their fathers and mothers, in terms of acceptance and control, compared to women abused by men who were not related to them. Furthermore, *incest victims who perceived their mothers negatively endorsed the promotion of autonomy in their attitudes toward child-rearing*.

The results were discussed in terms of:

1. Lack of positive parenting models when relationships with both parents are experienced as negative.
2. Conflicts of incest survivors regarding their early maturity.
3. The relationship of these findings to the tendency for intergenerational repetition of father-daughter incest.

The study by Schuetze P et al. [53] examined the association between child sexual abuse (CSA) and parenting outcomes, including parental stress, feelings of competence, and disciplinary strategies. It was hypothesized that maternal depression and current partner violence are mediators of the association between CSA, HSDD, and parenting.

The research participants were 263 first-time mothers, 107 with a history of CSA and 156 control mothers recruited from a prenatal clinic before the birth of their first child. The mothers were interviewed twice: once when they were between 28 and 32 weeks of gestation and again when their child was between 2 and 4 years old. During the first interview, women were asked about childhood experiences of sexual abuse. During their second interview, they were asked about current symptoms of pathology, experiences of partner violence, and parenting beliefs and practices.

The relationship between CSA and punitive discipline was mediated by maternal depression and current partner violence. CSA was associated with greater maternal depression and increased partner violence. CSA, maternal depression, and current partner violence were associated with more negative parenting perceptions and increased punitive discipline.

11.8 Conclusions

An individual's personal experiences during childhood and as a parent are likely key determinants of their subsequent parenting experiences. Child sexual abuse (CSA) is one of the most pathological experiences occurring in childhood and, therefore, may have a particularly likely impact on parental stress in the context of parenting one's own children. The research by Hugill M et al. [54] reviewed studies investigating the associations between previous CSA and subsequent parenting to determine the extent and consistency of effects, identify any mediators and moderators of the relationship, and assess the quality of the evidence base.

PsycINFO, Academic Search Complete, CINAHL, MEDLINE, Web of Science, PubMed, and PILOTS were the search engines of choice from the start date until March 4, 2016.

From this review, 14 studies met the inclusion criteria. Seven indicated a direct association between the experience of CSA and subsequent parental stress; two studies found no association; and five studies suggested that other variables such as locus of control and current stress factors may influence the relationship between CSA and parental stress. Additionally, ten studies suggested an indirect relationship between CSA and parental stress through the current level of depression. From this perspective, we could deduce that the investigation of hypoactive sexual desire disorder appears complex, heterogeneous, and intensely experienced by patients who report the discomfort.

An invitation to all doctors and psychosexual therapists; not to stop at appearances but to individually identify primary causes and developments in adulthood, as well as individual attempts to resolve the hypoactive sexual desire disorder. *We should ask ourselves: what does hypoactive desire signify in the clinical, psychological, and relational history of the individual patient?*

References

1. Tekin A, Meriç C, Sağbilge E, Kenar J, Yayla S, Özer ÖA, Karamustafalioğlu O. The relationship between childhood sexual/physical abuse and sexual dysfunction in patients with social anxiety disorder. Nord J Psychiatry. 2016;70(2):88–92. https://doi.org/10.3109/08039488.2015.1053097. Epub 2015 Jun 25. Erratum in: Nord J Psychiatry. 2016;70(5):399
2. Bruch MA, Heimberg RG. Differences in the perception of parental and personal characteristics between generalized and non-generalized social phobics. J Anxiety Disord. 1994;8:155–68.
3. Klonsky B, Dutton D, Liebel C. Developmental antecedents of private self-consciousness, public self-consciousness, and social anxiety. Genet Soc Gen Psychol Monogr. 1990;116:273–97.
4. Lieb R, Wittchen H, Hofler M, Fuetsch M, Stein M, Merikangas K. Parental psychopathology, parenting styles, and the risk of social phobia in offspring. Arch Gen Psychiatry. 2000;57:859–66.

5. Simon NM, Herlands NN, Marks EH, Mancini C, Letamendi A, Li Z, et al. Childhood maltreatment linked to greater symptom severity and poorer quality of life and function in social anxiety disorder. Depress Anxiety. 2009;26:1027–32.
6. Kuo JR, Goldin PR, Werner K, Heimberg RG, Gross JJ. Childhood trauma and current psychological functioning in adults with social anxiety disorder. J Anxiety Disord. 2011;25(4):467–73.
7. Bernstein D, Stein JA, Newcomb MD, Walker E, Pogge D, Ahluvalia T, et al. Development and validation of a brief screening version of the Childhood Trauma Questionnaire. Child Abuse Negl. 2003;27:169–90.
8. Mattick R, Clarke C. Development and validation of measures of social phobia, control fear, and social interaction anxiety. Behav Res Ther. 1998;36:455–70.
9. Spielberger CD, Gorsuch RL, Lushene RE. Manual for the state-trait anxiety inventory. Palo Alto, CA: Consulting Psychologists Press; 1970.
10. Coles ME, Gibb BE, Heimberg RG. Psychometric evaluation of the Beck Depression Inventory in adults with social anxiety disorder. Depress Anxiety. 2001;14:145–8. https://doi.org/10.1002/da.1057.
11. Walker EA, Gelfand A, Katon WJ, Koss MP, Von Korff M, Bernstein D, et al. Health status of women in adulthood with histories of childhood abuse and neglect. Am J Med. 1999;107:332–9.
12. Schulte-Herbrüggen O, Ahlers CJ, Kronsbein JM, Rüter A, Bahri S, Vater A, Roepke S. Impaired sexual function in patients with borderline personality disorder is determined by history of sexual abuse. J Sex Med. 2009;6(12):3356–63.
13. Sanchez DT, Kiefer AK. Body concerns inside and outside the bedroom: implications for sexual pleasure and problems. Arch Sex Behav. 2007;36:808–20.
14. Wiederman MW. Women's body image self-consciousness during physical intimacy with a partner. J Sex Res. 2000;37:60–8.
15. Pujols Y, Meston CM, Seal BN. The association between sexual satisfaction and body image in women. J Sex Med. 2010;7:905–16.
16. Sack M, Boroske-Leiner K, Lahmann C. Association of non-sexual and sexual trauma with body image and psychosomatic symptoms in psychosomatic outpatients. Gen Hosp Psychiatry. 2010;32:315–20.
17. Dyer AS, Feldmann RE Jr, Borgmann E. Body-related emotions in post-traumatic stress disorder following sexual abuse. J Child Sex Abus. 2015;24:627–40.
18. Finkelhor D, Browne A. The traumatic impact of child sexual abuse: a conceptualization. Am J Orthopsychiatry. 1985;55:530–41.
19. Rellini A. Review of empirical evidence for a theoretical model of understanding sexual problems in women with a history of CSA. J Sex Med. 2008;5:31–46.
20. Kilimnik CD, Meston CM. Role of body esteem in the sexual excitation and inhibition responses of women with and without a history of childhood sexual abuse. J Sex Med. 2016;13(11):1718–28.
21. Rellini AH, Hamilton LD, Delville Y, et al. Cortisol response during physiological sexual arousal in adult women with a history of childhood sexual abuse. J Trauma Stress. 2009;22:557–65.
22. Janssen E, Bancroft J. The psychophysiology of sex. Bloomington: Indiana University Press; 2007. The dual control model: the role of sexual inhibition and excitation in sexual arousal and behavior. p. 197–222.
23. Castellini G, LoSauro C, Lelli L, et al. Childhood sexual abuse moderates the relationship between sexual functioning and psychopathology of eating disorders in anorexia nervosa and bulimia nervosa: a 1-year follow-up study. J Sex Med. 2013;10:2190–200.
24. Dworkin E, Javdani S, Verona E, et al. Child sexual abuse and eating disorders: the mediating role of impulsive and compulsive tendencies. Psychol Viol. 2014;4:21–36.
25. Gray JA. A critique of Eysenck's theory of personality. In: Eysenck HJ, editor. A model of personality. Berlin: Springer-Verlag; 1981. p. 246–76.
26. Bigras N, Godbout N, Hébert M, Sabourin S. Cumulative adverse childhood experiences and sexual satisfaction in sex therapy patients: what role for symptom complexity? J Sex Med. 2017;14(3):444–54. https://doi.org/10.1016/j.jsxm.2017.01.013. Epub 2017 Feb 12

27. Tutino JS, Ouimet AJ, Shaughnessy K. How do psychological risk factors predict sexual outcomes? A comparison of four models of sexual outcomes in young women. J Sex Med. 2017;14:1232–40.
28. Rosen NO, Dubé JP, Corsini-Munt S, Muise A. Partners experience consequences, too: a comparison of the sexual, relational, and psychological adjustment of women with sexual interest/arousal disorder and their partners to control couples. J Sex Med. 2019;16(1):83–95.
29. Rosen NO, Corsini-Munt S, Dubé JP, Boudreau C, Muise A. Partner responses to low desire: associations with sexual, relational, and psychological well-being among couples coping with female sexual interest/arousal disorder. J Sex Med. 2020;17(11):2168–80.
30. Negriff S, Schneiderman JU, Smith C, Schreyer JK, Trickett PK. Characterization of sexual abuse experiences in young adolescents. Child Abuse Negl. 2014;38(2):261–70.
31. Breiding MJ. Prevalence and characteristics of sexual violence, stalking, and intimate partner violence victimization—National Intimate Partner and Sexual Violence Survey, United States, 2011. Am J Public Health. 2015;105(4):e11–2.
32. Johnson CF. Child sexual abuse. Lancet. 2004;364(9432):462–70.
33. Sable MR, Danis F, Mauzy DL, Gallagher SK. Barriers to reporting sexual assault for women and men: perspectives of college students. J Am Coll Heal. 2006;55(3):157–62.
34. Holmes WC. Male self-definitions of child sexual abuse experiences and potentially risky behavioral and psychiatric outcomes. Child Abuse Negl. 2008;32(1):83–97.
35. Paolucci EO, Genuis ML, Violato C. A meta-analysis of the published research on the effects of child sexual abuse. J Psychol. 2001;135(1):17–36.
36. Beck JJH, Bekker MD, van Driel MF, Roshani H, Putter H, Pelger RCM, et al. Prevalence of sexual abuse among patients seeking general urological care. J Sex Med. 2011;8(10):2733–8.
37. Warlick CA, Mathews R, Gerson AC. Keeping childhood sexual abuse on the urological radar screen. Urology. 2005;66(6):1143–9.
38. Kaliray P, Drife J. Childhood sexual abuse and subsequent gynecological conditions. Obstet Gynaecol. 2004;6(4):209–14.
39. Ellsworth P, Merguerian P, Copening M. Sexual abuse. J Urol. 1995;153:773–6.
40. Wijma B, Schei B, Swahnberg K, Hilden M, Offerdal K, Pikarinen U, et al. Emotional, physical, and sexual abuse in patients visiting gynecological clinics: a Nordic cross-sectional study. Lancet. 2003;361(9375):2107–13.
41. Beck J, Bekker M, Van Driel M, et al. Assessment of female sexual abuse in urological practice: results of a Dutch survey. J Sex Med. 2010;7:1464–8.
42. Peyronnet B, Mironska E, Chapple C, Cardozo L, Oelke M, Dmochowski R, et al. A comprehensive review of the pathophysiology of overactive bladder: paving the way for personalized treatment. Eur Urol. 2019;75(6):988–1000.
43. Danese A, McEwen BS. Adverse childhood experiences, allostasis, allostatic load, and age-related diseases. Physiol Behav. 2012;106(1):29–39.
44. Mayou R, Farmer A. Functional somatic symptoms and syndromes. BMJ. 2002;325(7358):265–8.
45. Owusu Sekyere E, Hardcastle T, Sathiram R, et al. Overview of lower urinary tract symptoms following intensive care unit admission for trauma. Afr J Urol. 2020;26:1–7.
46. Coyne KS, Wein AJ, Tubaro A, Sexton CC, Thompson CL, Kopp ZS, et al. The burden of lower urinary tract symptoms: assessing the impact of LUTS on health-related quality of life, anxiety, and depression: EpiLUTS. BJU Int. 2009;103(Suppl 3):4–11.
47. Breyer BN, Cohen BE, Bertenthal D, Rosen RC, Neylan TC, Seal KH. Lower urinary tract dysfunction in male Iraq and Afghanistan war veterans: association with mental health disorders: a population-based cohort study. Urology. 2014;83(2):312–9.
48. Epperson CN, Duffy KA, Johnson RL, Sammel MD, Newman DK. Lasting impact of childhood adversity on lower urinary tract symptoms in adult women. Neurourol Urodyn. 2020;39(5):1472–81.
49. Bae SM, Kang JM, Chang HY, Han W, Lee SH. PTSD is related to somatization in sexually abused children: the type of abuse moderates the effect of PTSD on somatization. PLoS One. 2018;13(6):e0199138.

50. Cour F, Robain G, Claudon B, Chartier-Kästler E. Childhood sexual abuse: how important is diagnosis for understanding and managing sexual, anorectal, and lower urinary tract symptoms. Prog Urol. 2013;23(9):780–92.
51. Cardozo L, Lange R, Voss S, Beardsworth A, Manning M, Viktrup L, et al. Short- and long-term efficacy and safety of duloxetine in women with predominant stress urinary incontinence. Curr Med Res Opin. 2010;26(2):253–61.
52. Marriage ND, Blackley AS, Panagiotaros K, Seklaoui SA, van den Bergh J, Hawkins R. Assessing parental understanding of sexualized behavior in children and adolescents. Child Abuse Negl. 2017;72:196–205.
53. Schuetze P, Eiden RD. The relationship between sexual abuse during childhood and parenting outcomes: modeling direct and indirect pathways. Child Abuse Negl. 2005;29(6):645–59.
54. Hugill M, Berry K, Fletcher I. The association between historical childhood sexual abuse and later parenting stress: a systematic review. Arch Womens Ment Health. 2017;20(2):257–71.

Borderline Personality, Couple's Relationship, and HSDD

12

Abstract

Borderline personality disorder (BPD) is a complex psychiatric disorder characterized by pervasive instability in emotional regulation, self-image, interpersonal relationships, and impulse control (Skodol et al., Biol Psychiatry. 51:951–63, 2002). Between 1% and 6% of adults meet the diagnostic criteria of the *Diagnostic and Statistical Manual of Mental Disorders*, fourth edition (DSM-IV) (Lenzenweger and Willett, J Abnorm Psychol. 116:684–700, 2007). BPD is the most common personality disorder among psychiatric patients, with a prevalence ranging from 10% in outpatient populations to 15%–25% in hospitalized patients (Gunderson, Am J Psychiatry. 166:530–9, 2009). BPD is associated with substantial mental and physical disabilities (Grant et al., J Clin Psychiatry. 69:533–45, 2008). Furthermore, BPD exhibits high and heterogeneous patterns of comorbidity with other psychiatric and substance abuse disorders (Eaton et al., Psychol Med. 41:1041–50, 2011), which are identified as strong and significant predictors of regular drinking before sex (Thompson et al., Drug Alcohol Depend. 141:167–70, 2014).

However, no study has examined the relationship between BPD and regular alcohol consumption before sex in the general population of the United States or other countries.

Keywords

NESARC · Borderline personality disorder · Drinking alcohol before sex · Risky sexual behaviors · Attachment · Conflict · Interpersonal functioning · Relationship quality · Relationship stability · Romantic relationships · Sexual fantasies · Paraphilias

E. V. Longhi, *Hypoactive Sexual Desire Disorder*,
https://doi.org/10.1007/978-3-032-00659-2_12

12.1 Introduction

The National Epidemiologic Survey on Alcohol and Related Conditions (NESARC) is a national survey in the United States [21] that collected data from 17,491 drinkers aged 18 years or older who were sexually active, had borderline personality disorder, and habitually drank alcohol before sex (mostly or always), residing in family or collective housing (*university residences, residential care centers, specialized nursing care facilities, group homes, military barracks, correctional institutions, worker dormitories, and facilities for homeless individuals).*

The in-person interviews of the first study were conducted in 2001–2002 with 43,093 respondents (response rate 81%). The second study was conducted in 2004–2005 with 34,653 participants (response rate 86.7%) [7].

The diagnostic interview used was *the Alcohol Use Disorder and Associated Disabilities Interview Schedule (AUDADIS-IV)* [8], *Wave 2 version* [9].

In fact, *the Alcohol Use Disorder and Associated Disabilities Schedule—Diagnostic and Statistical Manual of Mental Disorders, 4th edition (AUDADIS-IV), (DSM-IV)*—is a fully structured diagnostic interview designed to assess alcohol, drug, and mental disorders according to DSM-IV criteria in both clinical and general populations. The primary focus of AUDADIS-IV is measuring alcohol and drug use and associated disorders. Over the past 15 years, additional modules have been incorporated into AUDADIS-IV to assess a wide range of other psychiatric disorders and risk factors. Initially, in 1991–1992, AUDADIS-IV was used in a large-scale survey of the United States population, the National Longitudinal Alcohol Epidemiologic Survey of the National Institute on Alcohol Abuse and Alcoholism (NIAAA).

Since then, AUDADIS-IV has been used in the National Epidemiologic Survey on Alcohol and Related Conditions (NESARC) of the NIAAA (Wave 1 of 2001–2002, and in its 3-year follow-up Wave 2, conducted in 2004–2005).

One AUDADIS item concerned the frequency of alcohol intake before sex in the past year: "In the past year, how often have you drunk alcohol before having sex?". The possible answers were: never, rarely, sometimes, most of the time, and always.

AUDADIS items were used to operationalize the DSM-IV BPD criteria:

(i) Frantic efforts to avoid abandonment.
(ii) Pattern of unstable/intense relationships.
(iii) Disturbance of unstable self-image or self-identity.
(iv) Impulsivity in areas that are self-damaging.
(v) Recurrent suicidal behavior.
(vi) Affective instability or marked mood reactivity.
(vii) Chronic feelings of emptiness.
(viii) Inappropriate or intense anger.
(ix) Paranoia or transient stress-related dissociation.

To receive a diagnosis of BPD, participants needed to endorse five or more of these nine DSM-IV diagnostic criteria, with at least one causing social or occupational dysfunction.

Among sexually active drinkers, *the diagnosis of BPD was associated with a higher likelihood of regularly drinking before sex*. Of the nine diagnostic criteria for BPD, impulsivity in self-harming areas remained the only significant predictor of regular alcohol consumption before sex. Previous research has suggested complex, multidirectional associations between alcohol expectations, alcohol consumption, and sexual behaviors. Both acute intoxication and alcohol expectations contribute to risky sexual intentions and attitudes, increasing the likelihood of engaging in sexual intercourse when drinking [10].

12.2 Alcohol, Sex, HSDD, and Couple Relationship

The study by George WH et al. [11] sought to analyze the expectations of borderline patients regarding alcohol use to improve sexual performance. A total of 100 moderate male drinkers were evaluated. In a subsequent session, participants were led to believe they were consuming alcoholic or non-alcoholic beverages. In reality, no alcohol was administered. Each participant evaluated their own sexual arousal, rated a co-participant who was drinking alcohol or not on sexual disinhibition, and then viewed erotic slides with the co-participant. **The prophecy came true:** that expectations indirectly increased perceptions of sexual arousal and disinhibition. Sexual arousal, in turn, predicted perceived disinhibition, which then predicted the view.

The alcohol consumption of co-participants had direct and indirect effects on the view. Therefore, the role of alcohol in stimulating men's sexual response cannot be interpreted as if it occurred through a strictly pharmacological mechanism.

While HSDD seems to be present in borderline patients due to body dysmorphia, the inability to experience strong body sensations, obsessive behavior that anesthetizes the body map (as in bulimia *nervosa*), to the benefit of excessive eroticization.

The subsequent study by George WH et al. [12] then described four domains with reliable evidence of the effects of alcohol: sexualized social perceptions, sexual arousal, sexual risk-taking, and sexual aggression. Among the most relevant disorders of borderline personality (DP) is the marked impairment of relationships. The inability to pursue fundamental tasks of adult life, including "close and meaningful intimate relationships," is at the heart of the concept of personality disorder [13].

Some studies link personality pathology to the most extreme forms of maladaptive intimate relationships (partner violence); however, there is no study to date that examines more normative measures of marital functioning in relation to BPD characteristics.

The study by South SC et al. [14] examined the association between personality disorder symptoms and key characteristics of marital relationships, from satisfaction to verbal conflict and physical violence. Personality pathology is currently represented in the *DSM* as ten disorders that are presumably distinct from each other and from other forms of psychopathology, although they are grouped together in heterogeneous clusters: *(Cluster A—paranoid, schizoid, schizotypal, and dramatic); (Cluster B—antisocial, borderline, histrionic, narcissistic, and fearful); (Cluster C—avoidant, dependent, and obsessive-compulsive).*

It is hypothesized that each spouse's enduring vulnerabilities, including personality traits, influence both the stressful events that couples encounter and the types of behavioral exchanges that occur between spouses. In the last two decades, there has been a renewed interest in personality traits in relation to marital adjustment. This stems from several areas: a rebirth in the field of personality in general [15]; statistical advances that allow the examination of the joint influence and interdependence of couples on each other [16]; and the relatively modest and, at times, inconsistent associations found between marital functioning and more process-oriented interpersonal variables [17].

Among other things, a systematic review of the literature was conducted following the Preferred Reporting Items for Systematic Reviews and Meta-Analyses (PRISMA) guidelines [18].

Articles were retrieved through the electronic databases MEDLINE (National Library of Medicine–Bethesda USA) and PsycINFO, through two all-term searches for each of the two selected databases: the terms "*personality disorder*" and "*sexual dysfunction*." A second search strategy was performed on the same databases using the terms "*personality disorder*" and "Risky sexual behavior." The research period was from January 1, 2019 to April 25, 2022.

The database search identified 123 records. After removing 6 duplicates, 117 studies were examined by title and abstract. The screening process led to the exclusion of 101 studies. The full texts of the remaining studies were evaluated. Finally, 17 studies were included (published from January 1, 2019, to April 25, 2022).

Adan Sanchez et al. conducted [19] an assessment of the prevalence of high-risk sexual behaviors, (HRSB), their consequences, and associated factors in **103** young individuals attending a personality disorder clinic. Among these, a total of 77.7% were already sexually active, 37.5% did not use appropriate contraceptive methods, and 25.5% tested positive for a sexually transmitted infection. However, the study found no significant association between HRSB and clinical or demographic characteristics or symptom severity. **On the other hand**, an observational study conducted on **656** women aimed to *assess the association of self-reported pathological narcissistic traits with sexual functioning*. The results showed lower sexual functioning in individuals with vulnerable narcissistic traits, HSDD, and higher levels of body image self-awareness. Conversely, grandiose narcissistic traits appeared to be linked to higher levels of sexual functioning and lower self-awareness of body image [20].

Natoli and colleagues [21] studied the correlation between dependent personality profile and sexual relationships and activity. The work showed lower self-reported interpersonal dependency scores, HSDD, and higher healthy dependency scores in sexually active individuals and in individuals with past sexual activity.

Finally it was discovered [22] that psychotic spectrum disorders affect sexual functioning. While in some cases sexual symptoms can predict mental illnesses, the same link in BPD is not yet fully understood. However, the reduction in sexual health experienced in BPD should be considered in the evaluation of pre- or sub-clinical cases of psychotic spectrum disorders [23]. The transition to psychosis, in fact, could be predicted by various dysfunctional personality traits, such as schizotypy or paranoid ideation, which could influence sexual behavior [24].

12.3 Conclusion

To date, the evidence on Dissociative Personality Disorder (DPD) shows dysfunctional sexuality, as the fear of rejection from others can generate feelings of sexual failure and thus avoidance behaviors related to sexual experiences and HSDD. Indeed, Benotsch and colleagues described high levels of compromised sexual behaviors (such as having sex due to threats and fear of asking a partner to use a condom) in individuals with a marked dependency trait [25].

Lastly, to investigate the nature and frequency of sexual fantasies in psychiatric patients, the study by Colón Vilar G et al. [26] compared the frequency of four types of sexual fantasies across four different diagnoses of mood disorders and psychotic disorders, as well as three personality disorder groups.

The study participants included 133 psychiatric patients recruited from an urban hospital.

Sexual fantasies were compared among patients with schizophrenia, bipolar disorder, schizoaffective disorder, major depressive disorder, and three nonclinical samples drawn from the literature, then correlated with personality cluster scores.

Subjects were administered the *Structured Clinical Interview for DSM-IV Axis I* and *Axis II* disorders. Sexual fantasies were evaluated by the *Wilson Sexual Fantasies Questionnaire*, which measures four types of sexual fantasies: explorative, intimate, impersonal, and sadomasochistic.

Significant differences were found among the types of sexual fantasies, with subjects scoring higher in intimate sexual fantasies, and then explorative, impersonal, and sadomasochistic. No significant differences were found among the mood and psychotic diagnostic groups for any of the sexual fantasy scales, and the scores were within the normative range of the nonclinical samples.

Patients with high scores scored significantly higher on all four fantasy scales compared to those without. HSDD was reported by all patients through the lack of physical sensations. Drives such as erotic fantasies focused on eroticization and paraphilias.

References

1. Skodol AE, Siever LJ, Livesley WJ, Gunderson JG, Pfohl B, Widiger TA. Borderline II diagnosis: biology, genetics, and clinical course. Biol Psychiatry. 2002;51:951–63.

2. Lenzenweger MF, Willett JB. Predicting individual change in personality disorder characteristics through simultaneous individual change in personality dimensions linked to neurobehavioral systems: the longitudinal study of personality disorders. J Abnorm Psychol. 2007;116:684–700.
3. Gunderson JG. Borderline personality disorder: ontogenesis of a diagnosis. Am J Psychiatry. 2009;166:530–9.
4. Grant BF, Chou SP, Goldstein RB, et al. Prevalence, correlations, disability, and comorbidity of DSM-IV borderline personality disorder: results from the Wave 2 National Epidemiologic Survey on Alcohol and Related Conditions. J Clin Psychiatry. 2008;69:533–45.
5. Eaton NR, Krueger RF, Keyes KM, et al. Comorbidity of borderline personality disorder: relationship with the internalizing-externalizing structure of common mental disorders. Psychol Med. 2011;41:1041–50.
6. Thompson RG Jr, Eaton NR, Hu MC, Grant BF, Hasin DS. Regularly drinking alcohol before sex in the United States: effects of relationship status and alcohol use disorders. Drug Alcohol Depend. 2014;141:167–70.
7. Grant BF, Goldstein RB, Chou SP, et al. Sociodemographic and psychopathological predictors of first incidence of DSM-IV substance use, mood and anxiety disorders: results from the Wave 2 National Epidemiologic Survey on Alcohol and Related Conditions. Mol Psychiatry. 2009;14:1051–66.
8. Grant BF, Dawson DA, Hasin DS. The alcohol use disorder and associated disabilities interview schedule DSM-IV version. National Institute on Alcohol Abuse and Alcoholism website; [Accessed July 30, 2007]. http://www.niaaa.nih.gov.
9. Grant BF, Dawson DA, Hasin DS. The wave 2 National Epidemiologic Survey on alcohol and related conditions disorder and associated disabilities interview schedule DSM-IV version. Bethesda, MD: National Institute on Alcohol Abuse and Alcoholism; 2004.
10. George WH, Stoner SA. Understanding the acute effects of alcohol on sexual behavior. Annu Rev Sex Res. 2000;11:92–124.
11. George WH, Stoner SA, Norris J, Lopez PA, Lehman GL. Alcohol expectancies and sexuality: a self-fulfilling prophecy analysis of dyadic perceptions and behavior. J Stud Alcohol. 2000;61(1):168–76.
12. George WH, Blayney JA, Davis KC. Impact of acute alcohol consumption on sexuality: a look at psychological mechanisms. Annu Rev Clin Psychol. 2024;20(1):307–31.
13. Krueger RF, Skodol AE, Livesley WJ, Shrout PE, Huang Y. Synthesizing dimensional and categorical approaches to personality disorders: refining the research agenda for DSM-V Axis II. Int J Methods Psychiatr Res. 2007;16:65–73.
14. South SC, Turkheimer E, Oltmanns TF. Personality disorder symptoms and marital functioning. J Consult Clin Psychol. 2008;76(5):769–80.
15. Finanziatore DC. Personality. Annu Rev Psychol. 2001;52:197–221.
16. Campbell L, Kashy DA. Estimating actor, partner, and interaction effects for dyadic data using PROC MIXED and HLM: a user-friendly guide. Pers Relat. 2002;9:327–42.
17. Bradbury TN, Karney BR. Understanding and altering the longitudinal course of marriage. J Marriage Fam. 2004;66:862–79.
18. Page MJ, et al. The PRISMA 2020 statement: an updated guideline for reporting systematic reviews. BMJ. 2021;372:n71.
19. Adan Sanchez AY, et al. High-risk sexual behavior in young people with mental health disorders. Early Interv Psychiatry. 2019;13(4):867–73.
20. Pavanello Decaro S, et al. Narcissistic personality traits and sexual dysfunction in women: the role of self-awareness of body image. J Sex Med. 2021;18(11):1891–8.
21. Natoli AP, Schapiro-Halberstam S, Kolobukhova A. A multimethod investigation of sex, romantic relationships, and interpersonal dependency. Arch Sex Behav. 2021;50(6):2621–9.
22. Jannini TB, et al. Italian validation of the Arizona Sexual Experience Scale (ASEX) on patients affected by psychotic spectrum disorders. Riv Psichiatr. 2022;57(1):18–22.

23. Ciocca G, et al. Sexuality in subjects at ultra-high risk of psychosis and first-episode psychosis. A systematic review of the literature. Front Psychiatry. 2021;12:750033.
24. Ciocca G, et al. Sexuality in ultra-high risk individuals for psychosis and first-episode psychosis: a systematic review of the literature. Front Psych. 2021;12:750033.
25. Benotsch EG, et al. Addiction traits, relational power, and health risks in women receiving sexually transmitted infection clinic services. Behav Med. 2017;43(3):176–83.
26. Colón Vilar G, Concepción E, Galynker I, Tanis T, Ardalan F, Yaseen Z, Cohen LJ. Assessment of sexual fantasies in psychiatric inpatients with mood and psychotic disorders and comorbid personality disorder traits. J Sex Med. 2016;13(2):262–9.

Part IV

Specific Populations and Comorbidities

13 LGBT and Hypoactive Sexual Desire Disorder

Abstract

Relatively little is known about sexual dysfunction (SD) in men who have sex with other men (MSM). In 2004–2005, an internet sample of American MSM was recruited from gay-oriented networking, chat, and sexual news websites. The analytical sample included 7001 men aged 18 or older who reported having male sexual partners throughout their lives and having had oral or anal sex with a male partner in their most recent encounter in the past year (Mao J Sex Med 6:1378–1385, 2009). Overall, 79% of men reported one or more symptoms of SD in the past year, with **low sexual desire**, erection problems, and performance anxiety being the most common. Four distinct underlying patterns of sexual functioning were identified through LCA: low SD, erection/performance anxiety problems, low desire/pleasure, and high SD/sexual pain. High SD/sexual pain were distinguished from other patterns by the use of club drugs and the use of prescription and over-the-counter erectile dysfunction drugs before sex in the past year. In addition, men associated with the high SD/sexual pain group were younger, single, more likely to have poor mental and physical health, and more likely to have received a diagnosis of sexually transmitted infection in the past year compared to men in the no/low SD group (Hirshfield J Sex Med 7:3104–3114, 2010).

Keywords

LGBT and HSDD · Depression · HIV · Clinical studies with male LGBT patients · Sexual pain · HSDD research questionnaires in LGBT patients · PreP and sexually transmitted diseases · Drugs and alcohol

E. V. Longhi, *Hypoactive Sexual Desire Disorder*,
https://doi.org/10.1007/978-3-032-00659-2_13

13.1 Introduction

The 7001 patients recruited in the study by Hirshfield et al. [1] were recruited in 2004–2005 through an anonymous online survey. Eight American and Canadian gay-oriented websites—ranging from networking and sexual chat sites to news sites—hosted banners linking to the questionnaire on sexual behaviors, drug and alcohol consumption in the most recent encounter, and the previous year. Participants resided in every state of the United States, every Canadian province or territory, and abroad. The survey took between 10 and 15 minutes to complete, and no incentives were provided.

The analytical sample was limited to American men with male sexual partners in their lifetime and in the past year who were (at the time of the survey) sexually active with men.

13.2 The Research in Detail

Eleven percent of the analytical sample was excluded because they reported having had sexual relations also with women in the past year (202/262); 66% declared themselves bisexual, and 28% heterosexual.

The control group consisted of 174 patients who met the study's inclusion criteria, except for not having had sex with a man in the past year, with an average age of 44 years, were mostly white (80%) and had self-reported higher mental (52%) and physical (39%) health diagnoses in their lifetime than the men included in the analyses.

The study investigated whether there had been "a period of time" in the past 12 months during which SD symptoms occurred:

- Lack of interest in having sex (low sexual desire)
- Difficulty achieving or maintaining an erection (erection problems)
- Inability to have an orgasm (inability to reach orgasm)
- Anxiety, just before having sex, about the ability to perform sexually (performance anxiety)
- Reaching orgasm too quickly (premature ejaculation)
- Pain or discomfort during sex (pain during sex)
- Lack of pleasure during sexual intercourse, even if not painful (unenjoyable sex)

The seven questions from the research questionnaire were also used in MSM studies on SD symptoms in China and Australia [2]. The rates of self-reported sexual problems were high, with erectile dysfunction and lack of sexual desire being the most common. These high rates were consistent with limited data from previous Australian studies [3]. Men with more sexual problems were more likely to suffer from major depression ($P < 0.001$). A higher percentage of HIV-positive gay men (48.4%) reported more sexual problems compared to seronegative men (35.1%, $P = 0.002$). Factors independently associated with more sexual problems among seronegative gay men were poorer overall health and interpersonal isolation, whereas for HIV-positive gay men, they were the adoption of avoidance strategies to cope with everyday stress, engaging in sexual risks in casual encounters, and using antidepressants.

Returning to the study by Hirshfield S et al. 89% of men self-identified as homosexual, with 10% self-identifying as bisexual, and 1% as heterosexual. Among those who answered the question about HIV testing ($N = 6466$), 14% reported testing positive for HIV. HIV-positive men were significantly older than HIV-negative men (average difference, 3.9 years) and men not tested (average difference, 8.1 years). The prevalence of self-reported lifetime diagnoses—including mental and physical health factors—was as follows: hypoactive desire disorder (57%), anxiety (23%), depression (13%), bipolar disorder (5%), high cholesterol (17%), hypertension (13%), heart disease (3%), and diabetes (3%). There were linear associations between age and each physical health factor, as well as lifetime depression. The median number of male oral or anal sex partners in the past year ranged from 6 to 10, with 13% reporting any sexually transmitted infection (STI) in the past year.

About 79% of men reported having one or more symptoms of SD for "a period of time" in the past year. In order of prevalence, men reported:

- Low sexual desire (57%)
- Erection problems (45%)
- Performance anxiety (44%)
- Unenjoyable sex (37%)
- Inability to reach orgasm (36%)
- Premature ejaculation (34%)
- Pain during sex (14%)

The reporting of SD symptoms in the past year differed by some demographic and behavioral characteristics. Men under 30 years of age, with an income less than $50,000 [mostly HIV-positive patients, single, men who had used club drugs (25%), or erectile dysfunction drugs—prescription, (29%), non-prescription (16%)—before sex in the past year], men diagnosed with an STI (14%), and men with lifetime diagnoses of mental health problems (43%) or physical health problems (28%) were significantly more likely to have report SD and HSDD symptoms in the past year than their counterparts. Men who had fewer than six sexual partners in the past year were significantly less likely to report SD symptoms than men who reported more sexual partners.

In the past year, younger men were significantly more likely to report low sexual desire, premature ejaculation, pain during sex, and unenjoyable sex, compared to men aged 50 or older. Conversely, younger men were significantly less likely to report difficulty reaching orgasm, performance anxiety, or erection problems. Men aged 50 or older were more than twice as likely to have erection problems compared to men under 30 years of age. The symptoms of sexual dysfunction and hypoactive sexual desire disorder varied little by race, ethnicity, and income but varied based on HIV status and relationship status. HIV-positive men were significantly more likely than HIV-negative and untested men to report all of the previous year's sexual dysfunction symptoms, except for premature ejaculation. Compared to married or divorced, separated, or widowed men, single men were significantly more likely to report all of the previous year's sexual dysfunction symptoms, except for premature ejaculation and pain during sex.

The highest rates of hypoactive sexual desire disorder were associated with being younger, single, and having mental and physical health problems. The finding that young men reported low desire and poor or no sexual pleasure was surprising to researchers. However, little specific research has been conducted on low sexual desire in males [4].

Primary male hypoactive sexual desire disorder is rare and usually occurs in the context of a sexual secret, such as having a paraphilia, preferring masturbation to sex with others, having a history of sexual abuse, or experiencing an internal conflict about sexual identity [5]. Secondary hypoactive sexual desire disorder is more common and is often seen as a reaction to a sexual dysfunction, such as erectile dysfunction or premature ejaculation. It can stem from mental health problems (depression or anxiety), side effects of medications, or partner-related situations. Finally, the culture of "perfect sexual performance" can significantly contribute to secondary hypoactive sexual desire disorder.

It is important to remember that hypoactive sexual desire disorder in men is often misdiagnosed as erectile dysfunction due to the common prejudice that all men desire sex. This myth has led men not to seek treatment and has also resulted in misdiagnoses by healthcare providers. This may partly explain the failure rate of adequate treatment for erectile dysfunction. As part of an initial history and physical examination, a sexual history is necessary because most patients will not reveal any sexual problem unless explicitly asked. There are tests that exclusively concern sexual desire (Sexual Desire Inventory) and others have subscales for sexual desire (International Index of Erectile Function) [6].

13.3 HSDD and HIV-Positive Status

Using a cross-sectional survey model, Cove et al. [7] recruited a sample of 78 volunteer outpatient homosexual HIV-positive users who completed a self-assessment questionnaire. This tool examined sexual problems, perceived causes, and associated factors, including demographic data, health status, sexual behavior, self-justifications for taking sexual risks, and mood status (Hospital Anxiety and Depression Scale). Fifty (69%) of the 78 HIV-positive homosexual men reported one or more sexual problems. Erectile dysfunction (ED) was reported by 38%, increasing to 51% in the context of attempting to use a condom, along with hypoactive sexual desire disorder. A loss of interest in sex was reported by 41%, and 24% experienced delayed ejaculation.

The presence of sexual problems influenced condom use, as 33 (90%) of the 37 gay men with ED associated with condom use were inconsistent condom users in insertive sexual intercourse compared to 28% of those without this type of ED. The presence of ED did not reduce the frequency of anal intercourse, but those with condom-associated ED were significantly more likely to have engaged in receptive anal intercourse in the last 3 months (62%) compared to men without condom-associated ED (38%).

Risk cognitions—such as the desire to lose oneself in sex, leaving the responsibility of condom use to the active partner, and the perception *that condoms interfere with pleasure—were significantly more likely to be endorsed by those reporting condom-associated ED*. Other factors associated with sexual problems included low T cell counts. Psychological explanations were the most frequently cited causes of sexual problems, and hypoactive sexual desire disorder, both alone and in interaction with HIV disease itself and combination therapy. A high incidence of sexual problems was found in this sample of seropositive gay men.

Reducing unprotected anal intercourse in gay men infected with HIV is important to prevent further spread of this infection. Previous studies have shown that measure of personality traits—relevant to sexual excitability and the effects of anxiety—are correlated with unprotected anal intercourse in both gay and heterosexual men. Are HIV-positive gay men similar in this respect, or are there other personality-related factors that influence their sexual risk-taking?

This question [8] was addressed using a convenience sample of 156 HIV-positive gay men and 155 HIV-negative gay men, matched for age and unprotected anal intercourse risk. There were no significant differences between these two groups in measures of sexual excitability, inhibition of sexual arousal in risky situations, sensation seeking, and depression, propensity to anxiety or tendency toward increased sexual interest in negative mood states. HIV-positive men were, however, were more likely to report erectile problems and higher scores on a trait measure associated with inhibition of arousal due to the threat of performance failure and hypoactive sexual desire disorder. Such problems could be associated with reluctance to use condoms, thus increasing the likelihood of seroconversion and/or disease transmission. Alternatively, erectile problems could be a consequence of HIV infection. In either case, this has implications for prevention. The associations between HIV status, erectile problems, and unprotected anal intercourse need to be specifically addressed with individualized questionnaires and research protocols.

The study by **Dawson et al.** [9] collected saliva samples from *677* men who reported having had sex with other men in the previous 5 years, to assess how high-risk sexual behavior is influenced by awareness of partners' HIV serostatus among gay men.

Participants with an average age of 32.6 years, ranging from 16 to 71 years, were recruited from genitourinary medicine clinics and the gay community between March 1991 and April 1992. Fifty-two percent were from London, 21% from Manchester, 18% from central England, 6% from Bristol, and 3% from other areas.

Sixty-three percent had previously undergone a test for HIV antibodies. Ninety-four (16%) of the 580 satisfactory saliva samples tested for HIV-1 antibodies were seropositive; 17 men were not unaware of their HIV seropositive status.

The 577 men who reported having a sexual partner in the previous month provided information on 1380 partners during the period.

Forty-five percent of sexually active men reported engaging in some form of penetrative anal sex in the previous month, while 23% reported unprotected anal sex. However, HIV status was *known to both parties in only 15% of the 1380 partnerships*. Eight hundred and ninety-one partnerships did not involve penetrative anal sex, and 1107 involved only non-penetrative or penetrative sex always with a condom. Furthermore, 26% of partnerships involving unprotected penetrative anal sex involved mutual knowledge of HIV status, which was more likely to occur with regular partners than with non-regular or casual partners. Interestingly, 114 partners were known to be married, and 311 had an unknown marital status. A higher social class was associated with a reduced likelihood of engaging in risky sex, and high-risk sex was more common in partnerships where there was an age difference of more than 2 years.

Across these variations, the constant reported by patients was hypoactive sexual desire disorder in the last 5 years with same-sex partners.

13.4 Pre-Exposure Prophylaxis (PrEP) and Hypoactive Sexual Desire Disorder

Research investigating hypoactive sexual desire disorder in men who engage in sexual practices with other men also asked why sexually transmitted diseases are on the rise and whether PrEP has any impact on these diseases and on hypoactive sexual desire disorder. The emergence of PrEP as a strategy for HIV prevention has raised concerns that the intervention is exacerbating an already growing problem [10]. Like the "therapeutic optimism" of the late 1990s, PrEP could plausibly lead people to reduce condom use, increase the number of sexual partners, or change partners, thereby altering sexual networks in ways that could facilitate the transmission of STDs [11]. A study on the implementation of PrEP conducted in San Francisco, Washington DC, and Miami from 2012 to 2015 found that, although risky sexual behavior and STD rates remained stable after the start of PrEP, receptive anal sex without a condom increased among men in San Francisco, as did hypoactive sexual desire disorder [12]. Studies examining potential PrEP users regarding sexual behavior [13], including those undertaken before the widespread use of the intervention, have reported variable results. In some cases, these studies suggest that risk compensation occurred. A study on 180 HIV-negative MSM in New York City found that 35% of likely PrEP users indicated they would reduce condom use once on PrEP—a result also observed in Los Angeles—possibly reflecting fluctuating desire rather than a persistent change [14]. Using a mixed model, the study by Rotsaert et al. [15] explored attitudes of MSM PrEP users toward STDs, condoms, and condom use with non-stable partners to prevent STDs. They compared data from 22 in-depth interviews conducted at a large HIV/STD clinic between August 2021 and January 2022 and an online survey among 326 PrEP users between September 2020 and January 2022.

The themes identified in the qualitative data that influence decisions on condom use to prevent STDs were as follows: (1) awareness (e.g., perceived severity and susceptibility to STDs counseling), (2) motivation (e.g., concerns about STDs, sexual pleasure, and protection of one's health), and (3) perceived social norms and practices (e.g., reduced community-level condom use). Overall, 10.7% of respondents consistently used condoms with non-stable partners but also reported not having a stable sexual desire. Respondents who reported high or moderate levels of willingness to use condoms to prevent the acquisition of STDs were significantly more likely to use condoms for anal sex with non-stable partners; those who had started PrEP 6–12 months earlier were less likely to use condoms. The study found a wide variation in attitudes toward condom use for STD prevention among MSM using PrEP. It can be hypothesized that PrEP use may induce some patients into a "state of magical invulnerability" that leads them to risk anal intercourse with promiscuity and to overvalue condomless eroticism. The fact remains that HSDD remains a pathology often underlying these attempts at transgressive sexuality. PrEP and HSDD do not seem to be linked as a consequence of one another. However, PrEP has made it possible to ascertain that most patients have experienced or are experiencing HSDD in recent years of sexual practice. A sample of 78 volunteer outpatient HIV-positive homosexual users completed a self-assessment questionnaire in the study by Cove et al. [7]: here sexual problems, perceived causes, and associated factors were examined, including demographic data, health status, sexual behavior, self-justifications for taking sexual risks, and mood status (Hospital Anxiety and Depression Scale). Fifty (69%) of the 78 HIV-positive homosexual men reported one or more sexual problems. Erectile dysfunction (ED) was reported by 38%, increasing to 51% in the context of attempting to use a condom. The loss of interest in sex was reported by 41% and 24% experienced delayed ejaculation. The presence of sexual problems influenced condom use as 33 (90%) of the 37 gay men who had condom-associated ED were inconsistent condom users in sexual intercourse compared to 28% of those who did not have this type of ED. The presence of ED did not reduce the frequency of anal intercourse, but those with condom-associated ED were significantly more likely to have had receptive anal intercourse in the last 3 months (62%) compared to men without condom-associated ED (38%) ($P = 0.05$). Risk cognitions such as the desire to lose oneself in sex, leaving the responsibility for condom use to the active partner, and the perception that condoms interfere with pleasure were significantly more likely to be approved by those who reported erectile dysfunction with condoms.

A high incidence of sexual problems was found in this sample of HIV-positive gay men as was a high percentage of hypoactive sexual desire disorder (HSDD) often unspoken due to shame and feelings of inadequacy.

13.5 Conclusions

HSDD in men who have sex with other men is far from unusual, even though there is little scientific literature on the subject. There are more studies on homosexuality and the HIV-positive. The promiscuity of casual and group sexual behaviors also leads to other considerations.

Club drugs such as methylenedioxymethamphetamine (MDMA, ecstasy), gamma-hydroxybutyrate (GHB), and ketamine are among the fastest-growing drugs of abuse in the United States. Reports have shown that some gay and bisexual men are prone to using club drugs in a variety of settings. This is concerning since the use of club drugs has been linked to high-risk sexual behaviors. Moreover, the use of club drugs by HIV-positive individuals can have negative outcomes on disease progression, affecting adherence, causing pharmacological interactions with antiretrovirals, or potentially exacerbating immune suppression.

Participants at electronic dance music (EDM) events are a high-risk population for substance use and associated adverse effects. One study [16] examined substance use at EDM events, focusing on the associations between participation motives and substance use. Sociodemographic characteristics, event specifics, use in the past year, and participation motives were assessed through an online survey. The participants were 1345 attendees of Belgian EDM events (69.44% male, age $M = 22.63$, age $SD = 4.03$). Ecstasy, MDMA, Molly (52.28%), other synthetic hallucinogens (53.68%), ketamine (42.13%), amphetamines (40.45%), and alkyl nitrites (poppers) (32.76%) were most frequently used at festivals, outdoor, parties, and raves.

In nightclubs, cocaine (32.29%) was found to be prevalent, while other synthetic hallucinogens (15.79%) were consumed less often. At events with a more private character, cannabis (68.88%) and hallucinogenic mushrooms (66.44%) were used more frequently.

Apart from alcohol (47.76%), substance use in pubs and bars appeared negligible. It was shown that general enjoyment is the main reason for participation, followed by those related to music and socializing. A wide range of motives proved to be more important for users (dancing, exploration, escape, excitement, alcohol, drugs) compared to non-users, while some were associated with the use of specific substances. It was shown that the prevalence of substance use depends on the specifics of the environment. Moreover, the idea of a three-dimensional classification of the main motives for participating in music events was supported. Finally, correlations between participation motives and substance use, as well as specific substances, were estimated. The results could allow for more targeted approaches in prevention efforts and event management strategies.

Psychosexual therapy often applied or requested by people with homosexual sexual habits can be a valid approach to bring out co-causes of sexual, behavioral, and broader pathological dysfunctions. As well as proposing, together with other clinicians, a personalized approach to HSDD.

References

1. Hirshfield S, Chiasson MA, Wagmiller RL Jr, Remien RH, Humberstone M, Scheinmann R, Grov C. Sexual dysfunction in an internet sample of U.S. men who have sex with men. J Sex Med. 2010;7(9):3104–14.
2. Lau JT, Kim JH, Tsui HY. Prevalence and socio-cultural predictors of sexual dysfunction among Chinese men who have sex with men in Hong Kong. J Sex Med. 2008;5:2766–79.

3. Mao L, Newman CE, Kidd MR, Saltman DC, Rogers GD, Kippax SC. Self-reported sexual difficulties and their association with depression and other factors among gay men attending high HIV-caseload general practices in Australia. J Sex Med. 2009;6(5):1378–85.
4. McCarthy B, McDonald D. Evaluation, treatment, and relapse prevention: male hypoactive sexual desire disorder. J Sex Marital Ther. 2009;35:58–67.
5. Montgomery KA. Sexual desire disorders. Psychiatry (Edgmont). 2008;5:50–5.
6. O'Carroll R, Bancroft J. Testosterone therapy for low sexual interest and erectile dysfunction in men: a controlled study. Br J Psychiatry. 1984;145:146–51.
7. Cove J, Petrak J. Factors associated with sexual problems in HIV-positive gay men. Int J STD AIDS. 2004;15(11):732–6.
8. Bancroft J, Carnes L, Janssen E. Unprotected anal intercourse in HIV-positive and HIV-negative gay men: the relevance of sexual arousability, mood, sensation seeking, and erectile problems. Arch Sex Behav. 2005;34(3):299–305.
9. Dawson JM, Fitzpatrick RM, Reeves G, Boulton M, McLean J, Hart GJ, Brookes M. Awareness of sexual partners' HIV status as an influence upon high-risk sexual behaviour among gay men. AIDS. 1994;8(6):837–41.
10. Grant RM, Lama JR, Anderson PL, McMahan V, Liu AY, Vargas L, et al. Pre-exposure chemoprophylaxis for HIV prevention in men who have sex with men. N Engl J Med. 2010;363:2587–99.
11. McCormack S, Dunn DT, Desai M, Dolling DI, Gafos M, Gilson R, et al. Pre-exposure prophylaxis to prevent the acquisition of HIV-1 infection (PROUD): efficacy results from the pilot phase of a pragmatic open-label randomised trial. Lancet. 2016;387:53–60.
12. Liu AY, Cohen SE, Vittinghoff E, Anderson PL, Doblecki-Lewis S, Bacon O, et al. Pre-exposure prophylaxis for HIV infection integrated with municipal and community-based health services. JAMA Intern Med. 2016;176:75–84.
13. Hoff CC, Chakravarty D, Bircher AE, Campbell CK, Grisham K, Neilands TB, et al. Attitudes towards PrEP and intended condom use among HIV-negative and HIV-discordant male couples. AIDS Patient Care STDs. 2015;29:408–17.
14. Brooks RA, Landovitz RJ, Kaplan RL, Lieber E, Lee SJ, Barkley TW. Risk sexual behaviors and acceptability of HIV pre-exposure prophylaxis among HIV-negative gay and bisexual men in serodiscordant relationships: a mixed-methods study. AIDS Patient Care STDs. 2012;26:87–94.
15. Rotsaert A, Nöstlinger C, Van Landeghem E, Vanbaelen T, Wouters E, Buffel V, Scheerder G, Schim van der Loeff M, Vuylsteke B, Reyniers T. Pre-exposure prophylaxis users' attitudes about sexually transmitted infections and its influence on condom use: a mixed-method study in Belgium. AIDS Patient Care STDs. 2022;36(12):483–92.
16. Van Dyck E, Ponnet K, Van Havere T, Hauspie B, Dirkx N, Schrooten J, Waldron J, Grabski M, Freeman TP, Curran HV, De Neve J. Substance use and attendance motives of electronic dance music (EDM) event attendees: a survey study. Int J Environ Res Public Health. 2023;20(3):1821.

Hypoactive Sexual Desire Disorder in Transgender Patients

14

Abstract

Hypoactive sexual desire disorder (HSDD) is a common condition among transgender women. However, to date, there are no specific guidelines for managing HSDD in transgender individuals. Clinically relevant publications on the management of HSDD (from 1985 to 2020) were searched in the *PubMed* and *Medline databases*, using the following terms: "sexual desire," "sexual health," "HSDD," "transgender," "gender affirmation treatment," "sexual therapy," "testosterone treatment," "central nervous system active drugs," and variants. Since sexual desire may be influenced by various factors, a comprehensive evaluation of HSDD should include biological, psychological, and social factors, in order to identify possible predisposing, precipitating, and maintaining factors. Among treatment options, transgender women may benefit from various sexual therapy strategies, and or central nervous system active drugs, such as *flibanserin*, bremelanotide, bupropion, and buspirone, and transdermal testosterone, bearing in mind that this option may be poorly accepted by patients due to the risk of virilizing effects (Cocchetti et al. Int J Impot Res 33:703–709, 2020).

Keywords

HSDD in transgender patients · GCT · Hormonal treatment · Sexual fantasies · Central nervous system active drugs · Sexual health · HIV · Gender-affirming care · Binary gender system · Hormone replacement therapy (HRT) · Postoperative pain · Transgender issues (GLBT) · PHQ-9 · Gender reassignment procedures · Major depressive disorder

E. V. Longhi, *Hypoactive Sexual Desire Disorder*,
https://doi.org/10.1007/978-3-032-00659-2_14

14.1 Introduction

Two factors that are likely associated with the sexual experiences of transgender individuals are their psychological well-being and body satisfaction. There are several indications that dissatisfaction with one's appearance or feelings of gender dysphoria can make it more difficult to enjoy or be satisfied with sexual experiences.

Furthermore, although transgender individuals generally report improved sexual satisfaction after hormonal treatment or genital surgery to modify sexual characteristics (GCT), the results also indicate that satisfaction with one's genitals plays a significant role in sexual satisfaction after GCT [2].

Since psychological well-being and body satisfaction can vary greatly among groups of transgender individuals with different treatment desires, it is essential to explore the role of these factors in their sexual experiences.

For many trans individuals, being trans and the transition process profoundly influence the way they subjectively experience sexuality in the broadest sense of the term.

Existing research on the sexuality of trans individuals often does not focus on the subjective level of experience. It mostly addresses sexuality to uncover pathologies that are said to guide trans identity, the risk of HIV transmission, or sociocultural norms on gender and sexual identity.

14.2 Clinical Research Paradigms

The theory and research [3] on the topic of autogynephilia, for example, aimed not so much at describing the sexual experience of male-to-female (MtF) individuals but rather at describing or testing the theory of autogynephilia as an explanation for their desire to transition. Similarly, the identity development of gay and bisexual female-to-male (FtM) individuals was studied to determine whether these individuals' cross-gender identity was "bona fide," [3] as homosexuality after transition was a contraindication to sex reassignment therapy (SRT) [4].

Recently, however, more research has explicitly aimed to study the sexual functioning and experiences of trans individuals. For example, there has been an increase in research investigating the relationships between hormone replacement therapy (HRT), sex-reassignment surgery (SRS), sexual satisfaction, and sexual health [5].

This more recent medical research provides relevant information on overall sexual functioning, although it is less informative about the subjective experience of sexuality among trans individuals. Moreover, it only includes clinical samples of trans individuals who have been diagnosed with a gender identity disorder and who have undergone sex-reassignment/realignment procedures.

In a recent study of 237 Swedish trans individuals, a broader range of individuals was included, and subjective evaluations of sexual experience, attitudes, and the need for information and interventions in the area of sexual health were addressed. Although the survey design did not allow for an in-depth exploration of these topics, this study provides interesting guidelines for further research.

Research on the sexuality of trans individuals seems to be shifting from using sexuality as an indirect measure to address other topics to identifying sexual experiences as a central concern [6].

Returning to the study by Doorduin et al. [2], interviews with transgender patients, lasting on average 2 hours and 45 minutes, with a range from 1 hour and 12 minutes to 2 hours and 56 minutes, were conducted, recorded and transcribed with the individuals' permission.

The questions explored sexual preferences and identity, sexual and romantic relationships, sex with other people, masturbation, sexual fantasies, taste for pornography and eroticism, bodily experiences, sexual functioning, communication about sex, the meaning of sexuality for the participant, the role of being trans in relation to sexuality, and future expectations for themselves regarding sex and sexuality.

All participants in this study experienced or had experienced ***feelings of incongruity between gender identity, gender embodiment, and or social perception of gender to some extent during their lives. The extent and intensity of these feelings varied among participants. Feelings of incongruity increased after coming out and during the transition process, while they decreased or disappeared during the transition.***

Since bodily experience and social perceptions of gender were intertwined with experiences of sexuality, these feelings of incongruity negatively affected the participants' sexual pleasure. Sex was experienced as a part of life where these feelings were particularly present.

For some participants, it was mainly their body that was "in the way"; for others, the social perception of gender or the incongruity of the gender role was more evident.

Some participants reported, in addition to HSDD, a general lack of control over their body's physical reaction to sexual stimuli, feeling that their body's sexual arousal or orgasm were involuntary, and they also noticed a lack of control over their partners' sexual touches. Two FtM participants indicated that sex with their partner before coming out evoked the feeling of having been raped.

14.3 Sexuality After Treatment

Participants who underwent hormonal and/or surgical treatments related to their gender transition reported that their sexual functioning changed during these periods.

Four MtF participants and five FtM participants reported experiences with hormone replacement therapy. ***Participants from both groups described changes in their sexual desire, arousal, sensitivity of sexual organs, and orgasm. All MtF participants reported a decrease (initial) or loss of sexual desire and difficulty maintaining sexual arousal.***

Two participants who reported being on hormone replacement therapy for the longest period described an eventual increase or return of their desire after starting hormone replacement therapy. All FtM participants on hormone replacement therapy, except one, reported an initial increase in sexual desire and arousal. *In one case, this desire subsequently decreased or returned to the level of desire experienced before hormone replacement therapy.*

Regarding sexual fantasies between sexes, it is notable that this topic has received much attention in clinical research but lacks an inductive empirical approach. Perhaps what plays a role is that descriptions of this practice by trans people have been viewed with suspicion by some proponents of "autogynephilia" theories.

A follow-up study [7] **was also** conducted on 55 transsexual patients (32 male-to-female and 23 female-to-male) who underwent sex reassignment surgery (SRS) to assess the outcome of sexual and overall health. Although all male-to-female treated continuously with estrogens, had total testosterone levels within the normal female range due to the effects of estrogens on sex hormone-binding globulin, only 32.1% achieved normal levels of free testosterone.

After SRS, the transsexual person's expectations were met at an emotional and social level, but less so at a physical and sexual level, although a large number of transsexuals (80%) reported an improvement in their sexuality.

Female-to-male participants masturbated significantly more frequently than male-to-female participants, and in the female-to-male group, there was a trend toward greater sexual satisfaction, greater sexual arousal, and easier achievement of orgasm. Most participants reported a change in orgasmic sensation—toward a more powerful and brief sensation for female-to-male and more intense, smoother, and longer for male-to-female participants.

Over two-thirds of male-to-female participants reported the secretion of a vaginal fluid during sexual arousal, coming from the Cowper's glands, left in place during surgery. In female-to-male participants with erectile prostheses, sexual expectations were more fully realized (compared to those without), but pain during intercourse was reported more often.

Among all these results, HSDD was evident during either permanent or fluctuating periods.

With regard to vaginoplasty, the procedure is performed to create an aesthetic and functional vulva and vaginal canal that allow for receptive intercourse, an erogenous sensation of the clitoris, and a downward urine flow. Penile inversion vaginoplasty (PIV) is a single surgical procedure that involves the rearrangement of the anatomical components of the penis and the scrotum, allowing many patients to achieve these anatomical goals.

Other options include minimal depth, peritoneal, and intestinal vaginoplasty. It has been shown that patients' quality of life improves dramatically after vaginoplasty, but complication rates can reach 70%.

Fortunately, most complications do not alter the long-term postoperative clinical outcomes and can be managed without surgery during the acute perioperative phase. However, significant complications—such as rectal injuries, rectovaginal fistulas, and urethral or introital stenosis—can substantially affect the patient's experience. *Hence, persistent HSDD.*

Innovations in approaches and surgical techniques have shown promising initial results for reducing complications and increasing vaginal depth, but long-term data are scarce.

The study by BOAS et al. [8] conducted a retrospective review of the clinical records of a single surgeon's experience with penile inversion vaginoplasty, with or without revision labiaplasty and/or clitoroplasty between *July 2014 and June 2016* in a cohort of gender-diverse patients assigned male at birth. Demographic data, complications, and patient quality-of-life data were collected. Univariate and multivariate comparisons were completed.

One hundred and seventeen patients underwent penile inversion vaginoplasty. Of these, **28** patients (23.9%) underwent revision labiaplasty and/or clitoroplasty, with nine patients (7.7%) undergoing both procedures. Patients undergoing penile inversion vaginoplasty that required revision were significantly more likely to have granulation tissue, intravaginal scarring, and complete vaginal stenosis. Most patients undergoing revision labiaplasty and/or clitoroplasty reported satisfaction with the final surgical outcome (82.4%) and resolution of genital-related dysphoria (76.5%) but also experienced fluctuating or worsening HSDD.

However, there is little literature that synthesizes urinary complications after PIV surgery, and it is necessary to compile these complications to advise patients before and after surgery on managing surgical expectations. In this systematic review, we summarize the prevalence of urinary complications after PIV.

The study by Ding et al. [9] conducted research in the *MEDLINE*, *EMBASE*, *CINAHL*, and Scopus databases in July 2020. *The primary outcome was the prevalence of urinary and surgical complications in patients after penile inversion vaginoplasty*. The aggregate prevalence was determined from extrapolated data.

The **ROBINS-I** tool was used to assess the quality of the study. The study was prospectively registered on **PROSPERO** (CRD 42020204139).

Of 843 unique records, 27 articles were grouped for the synthesis, with **3388** patients. Overall patient satisfaction ranged from 80% to 100%. The most common urological complications included poor or divergent stream (11.7%), meatal stenosis (6.9%), and irritative symptoms (frequency, urgency, nocturia) (11.5%). Other urinary complications included retention requiring catheterization (5.1%), incontinence (8.7%) urethral stenosis (4.6%), and urinary tract infection (5.6%).

14.4 HSDD and Pain

A team of scholars met periodically via a Zoom conference between *April 2021 and February 2023* to discuss relevant literature with the aim of providing an overview on the incidence, phenotype, and mechanisms of pain in transgender patients [10].

Review sections were written after gathering information from systematic searches of the electronic literature published or available to the public to compile for publication as part of a thematic series on gender and pain in *Frontiers in Pain Research*.

Although transgender individuals represent a significant and increasingly visible component of the population, many researchers and physicians are not well informed about the diversity of gender identity, physiology, hormonal status, and medical procedures for gender affirmation used by transgender patients and other gender diverse individuals.

Both transgender and cisgender individuals have many of the same medical concerns, but the research and treatment of these medical needs must reflect an understanding of how sex differences, gender, gender affirmation medical procedures, and minority status influence pain.

Of particular importance is the need for extensive, long-term follow-up studies to ascertain the best practices for such procedures. A multidisciplinary approach with personalized interventions is by far the most scientifically supported hypothesis.

14.5 Conclusions

An unknown percentage of transsexual women (defined as post-operative male-to-female transsexuals undergoing estrogen replacement therapy) suffer from hypoactive sexual desire disorder (HSDD). It has been suggested that the absence of ovarian androgen production together with increased levels of sex hormone-binding globulin (SHBG) related to estrogen treatment, could lead to HSDD due to low levels of biologically available testosterone.

A cross-sectional study [11] recruited 62 transsexual women and 30 patients in an ovulating control group. Questionnaires measuring sexual desire (sexual desire inventory) and sexual and relational satisfaction (Maudsley Marital Questionnaire) were completed. Serum levels of total testosterone, (LH), and SHBG were measured in random blood samples obtained from transsexual women and in the early follicular phase in ovulating women.

The transsexual group had lower levels of total and calculated free testosterone compared to ovulating women. HSDD was reported in 34% of transsexual women and 23% of ovulating women. Both groups reported similar levels of sexual desire. For transsexual women, no significant correlation was found between sexual desire and total or free testosterone. In ovulating women, these correlations were significant.

HSDD is reported in a third of transsexual women.

This prevalence is not substantially different from controls, despite significantly lower levels of free testosterone, which argues against a significant role of testosterone in this specific group.

Finally, although many studies have shown that transgender women (TW) tend to have more depressive symptoms compared to the general population, the exact prevalence of major depressive disorder and the risk factors contributing to it have not yet been studied, especially in those who have undergone gender affirmation genital surgery (GAS).

Every TW aged between 20 and 60 years attending the Thai Red Cross transgender clinics for a postoperative check-up was invited to complete a self-assessment questionnaire, including demographic data, the Thai Patient Health Questionnaire 9 (PHQ-9), satisfaction with psychosocial factors (family, friends, and society relationships), sexual experiences, and outcomes of gender affirmation treatments before and after GAS, and finally, factors contributing to depressive symptoms [12].

Correlations between demographic data and depressive scores were tested. The paired t-test was used to compare pre and post GAS data.

A total of 97 TW were analyzed, with 22.7% considered to have "major depression" (PHQ-9 $\geq$ 9) after GAS. Postoperative improvements were observed in satisfaction with psychosocial factors and outcomes of gender affirmation treatment, particularly in sexual experience.

It was found that the severity of depression was negatively correlated with age and sexual satisfaction and HSDD. In particular, the presence of masculine features before surgery, poor social support and understanding, and postoperative surgical complications were widely considered factors contributing to depressive symptoms.

Compared to non-GAS TW, depression among those who underwent GAS in Thailand was lower but still significant and was linked to a younger age and poor postoperative sexual experiences. These findings were supported by the number of qualitative assessments in the psychosexual domain and postoperative treatment outcomes.

Appendix

A study by Tordoff et al. [13] recruited **104** youths aged between 13 and 20 years: **63** transmasculine individuals (60.6%), **27** transfeminine individuals (26.0%), **10** non-binary or gender fluid individuals (9.6%) and four young people who answered "I don't know" or did not answer the question on gender identity (3.8%).

At the beginning, 59 individuals (56.7%) suffered from moderate to severe depression, 52 individuals (50.0%) suffered from moderate to severe anxiety, and 45 individuals (43.3%) reported self-harm or suicidal thoughts.

At the end of the study, 69 young people (66.3%) had received PB, GAH, or both interventions, while 35 young people had not received either of the two interventions (33.7%). After adjusting for temporal trends and potential confounding factors, it was observed that there was a 60% lower rate of depression and a 73% lower likelihood of suicidality among young people who had started PB or GAH compared to young people who had not started them.

The mental health outcomes of interest were assessed using the Patient Health Questionnaire 9-item (PHQ-9) and Generalized Anxiety Disorder 7-item (GAD-7) scales, which were dichotomized into measures of moderate or severe depression and anxiety, respectively. Any self-report of self-harm or suicidal thoughts in the previous 2 weeks was assessed using question 9 of the PHQ-9. Generalized estimating equations were used to evaluate the change from baseline in each outcome at 3, 6, and 12 months of follow-up.

References

1. Cocchetti C, Ristori J, Mazzoli F, Vignozzi L, Maggi M, Fisher AD. Management of hypoactive sexual desire disorder in transgender women: a guide for clinicians. Int J Impot Res. 2020;33(7):703–9.
2. Doorduin T, van Berlo W. Trans people's experience of sexuality in The Netherlands: a pilot study. J Homosex. 2014;61(5):654–72. https://doi.org/10.1080/00918369.2014.865482.
3. Lawrence AA. Autogynephilia: a paraphilic model of gender identity disorder. J Gay Lesbian Psychother. 2004;8(1/2):69–87.
4. Coleman E, Bockting W, Gooren L. Homosexual and bisexual identity in sex-reassigned female-to-male transsexuals. Arch Sex Behav. 1993;22(1):37–50.
5. Wierckx K, Elaut E, Van Caenegem E, Van De Peer F, Dedecker D, Van Houdenhove E, T'Sjoen G. Sexual desire in female-to-male transsexual persons: exploration of the role of testosterone administration. Eur J Endocrinol. 2011;165(2):331–7.
6. Gäredal M, Orre C. "Feeling safe turns me on!": a study on trans people's experiences and thoughts about sex and the need for knowledge and interventions regarding sexual health. RFSL & RFSL Ungdom; 2011.
7. De Cuypere G, T'Sjoen G, Beerten R, Selvaggi G, De Sutter P, Hoebeke P, Monstrey S, Vansteenwegen A, Rubens R. Sexual and physical health after sex reassignment surgery. Arch Sex Behav. 2005;34(6):679–90.
8. Boas SR, Ascha M, Morrison SD, Massie JP, Nolan IT, Shen JK, Vyas KS, Satterwhite T. Outcomes and predictors of revision labiaplasty and clitoroplasty after gender-affirming genital surgery. Plast Reconstr Surg. 2019;144(6):1451–61.
9. Ding C, Khondker A, Goldenberg MG, Kwong JCC, Lajkosz K, Potter E, Millman A, Krakowsky Y, Perlis N. Urinary complications after penile inversion vaginoplasty in transgender women systematic review and meta-analysis. Can Urol Assoc J. 2023;17(4):121–8.
10. Anger JT, Case LK, Baranowski AP, Berger A, Craft RM, Damitz LA, Gabriel R, Harrison T, Kaptein K, Lee S, Murphy AZ, Said E, Smith SA, Thomas DA, Valdés Hernández MDC, Trasvina V, Wesselmann U, Yaksh TL. Pain mechanisms in transgender individuals: a review. Front Pain Res (Lausanne). 2024;5:1241015.
11. Elaut E, De Cuypere G, De Sutter P, Gijs L, Van Trotsenburg M, Heylens G, Kaufman JM, Rubens R, T'Sjoen G. Hypoactive sexual desire in transsexual women: prevalence and association with testosterone levels. Eur J Endocrinol. 2008;158(3):393–9.
12. Nimitpanya P, Wainipitapong S, Wiwattarangkul T, Suwan A, Phanuphak N, Panyakhamlerd K. Evaluation of mental health and satisfaction following transfeminine gender-affirming surgery in Thailand. Transgend Health. 2022;7(1):61–7.
13. Tordoff DM, Wanta JW, Collin A, Stepney C, Inwards-Breland DJ, Ahrens K. Mental health outcomes in transgender and nonbinary youths receiving gender-affirming care. JAMA Netw Open. 2022;5(2):e220978.

HSDD in Cancer Patients

15

Abstract

As survival rates for women and men diagnosed with cancer continue to improve, sexual dysfunction, including low sexual desire, is becoming more prevalent. It has been shown that a cancer diagnosis, treatment, and treatment-induced changes affect sexual desire in all patients. Understanding low sexual desire and current treatment options will allow physicians to effectively address it, enabling better quality of life for all patients.

Keywords

Breast cancer · DSM-IV · Sexual dysfunction · Sexuality · Aromatase inhibitor · BRCA1/2 · Mastectomy · Risk-reducing salpingo-oophorectomy · Sexuality · Tamoxifen, couples · Dyadic research · Psychological distress · Rectal cancer · Relational satisfaction · Sexual functioning · Help-seeking behavior · Male · Prostate cancer · Prostate neoplasms · Psycho-oncology and psychosexology · Adolescent and young adult (AYA) cancer

15.1 Introduction

Investigating variations in the quality of life among cancer patients, the study by Luo F et al. [1] evaluated the literature regarding the prevalence, predictive factors, and current treatments for sexual hypoactive sexual desire disorder in patients who have experienced a diagnosis of breast cancer.

A search was conducted through the *PubMed* search engine, selecting English-language articles in peer-reviewed journals published between 2005 and 2021. The keywords used were: *"breast cancer" and "sexual function," "sexual dysfunction," "hypoactive sexual desire disorder," "sexual drive," or "sexual desire."* Articles presenting a study or survey evaluating sexual drive in breast cancer survivors or patients, its identification, management, or treatment were examined.

E. V. Longhi, *Hypoactive Sexual Desire Disorder*,
https://doi.org/10.1007/978-3-032-00659-2_15

A total of **37 studies** evaluating the relationship between breast cancer, its treatments, and the effects induced by the chosen treatment for breast cancer and sexual desire were included. *The studies indicated that hypoactive sexual desire disorder persisted throughout the timeline from breast cancer diagnosis to post-treatment.* Surgical treatment, body image, and adjuvant hormonal therapy appeared to be some of the factors influencing low sexual desire in breast cancer survivors. Treatment options included nonpharmacological, pharmacological, and hormonal therapies.

15.1.1 Partner Reactions

The study by Hummer SB et al. [2] also evaluated the impact of HSDD on the partners of breast cancer patients; reference was made to the *Diagnostic and Statistical Manual of Mental Disorders, 4th edition* (DSM-IV).

Baseline data from a study on the efficacy of online cognitive-behavioral therapy for HSDD in patients diagnosed with breast cancer were collected and evaluated. The women completed self-report questionnaires to assess sexual functioning, sexual distress, relational intimacy, marital functioning, menopausal symptoms, body image, and psychological distress. Their partners completed questionnaires to assess sexual functioning.

The study included **169 breast cancer diagnosed patients and 67 partners**.

The most common female sexual dysfunctions were hypoactive sexual desire disorder (HSDD; 83%), sexual arousal disorder (40%), and dyspareunia (33%). Endocrine therapy was associated with HSDD and immunotherapy was associated with dyspareunia. Advanced age was associated with less sexual distress ($P < 0.001$). Depressive symptoms were higher in patients with sexual arousal disorder.

An indication for erectile disorder was present in two-thirds of partners. The lower overall sexual satisfaction of the partner was associated with lower overall sexual functionality of breast cancer diagnosed patients, lower female arousal, and lower female sexual satisfaction. Less vigorous male erectile function was correlated with greater female sexual pain. The partners of women who underwent breast reconstruction reported slightly better orgasmic function and overall sexual function compared to the partners of women who underwent conservative breast treatment.

In practice, endocrine therapy and immunotherapy are significant risk factors for hypoactive sexual desire disorder **(HSDD) and dyspareunia** in patients diagnosed with breast cancer. *Hence, it is crucial to involve both partners in sexual counseling following breast cancer treatment.*

The prevalence of sexual dysfunction in women with a history of breast cancer *following risk-reducing salpingo-oophorectomy (RRSO) was the focus of research by TUCKER PE* et al. [3], *primarily on the impact on sexuality. A secondary objective was to examine the effect of a previous breast cancer diagnosis and other factors on sexuality and quality of life (QoL) outcomes. This is a cross-sectional study of 119 women who underwent RRSO between 2009 and 2014. Data were collected* *through a questionnaire including demographic information and validated measures of sexual function, sexual distress, relationship satisfaction, body image, psychological stress, symptoms of post-surgical menopause, and overall quality of life.*

Sixty of the 119 participants who underwent RRSO had a history of breast cancer. Eighty percent of the women with breast cancer had female sexual dysfunction (FSD), and 82% had hypoactive sexual desire disorder (HSDD) after RRSO. Bilateral mastectomy was associated with higher rates of HSDD and greater body image self-consciousness (BISC) during sexual activity. Breast reconstruction was associated with higher relationship satisfaction scores (RAS). Compared to tamoxifen, aromatase inhibitors (AI) were significantly associated with reduced lubrication, arousal, and orgasm, and increased dyspareunia. A previous diagnosis of breast cancer was not associated with the prevalence of FSD.

15.1.2 Hysterectomy, HSDD, Surgical Menopause

Sexual well-being is an essential component of a woman's quality of life to maintain an active sex life; therefore, before planning any surgical intervention, including hysterectomy and bilateral salpingo-oophorectomy, the emotional and relational cost of surgery should be evaluated. About 75% of all hysterectomies are performed together with bilateral salpingo-oophorectomy for benign gynecological diseases [4]. *Several studies have investigated the effects of surgical menopause on women's sex lives and have found conflicting results. Some researchers have found negative impacts of surgical menopause on sexual functions, while others have indicated that it had no effect or even improved sexual life* [5, 6].

The study by Bıldırcın FD et al. [7] *included 151 women with surgical menopause (SM), 357 women with natural menopause (NM), and 186 women in perimenopause (PM), all of whom attended menopause and gynecology clinics at the Ondokuz Mayis University Department of Obstetrics and Gynecology in Samsun, Turkey, between 2007 and 2017. All authors and the study protocol complied with the World Medical Association's Helsinki Declaration on ethical issues and principles in research involving human subjects. Local ethical committee approval (Ondokuz Mayis University Clinical Research Ethics Committee) for the study (OMU-KAEK 2013/298) was obtained, and written informed consent was obtained from the subjects who participated.*

Menopausal participants were aged between 49 and 62 years and had been postmenopausal for at least 1 year. Women with surgical menopause (SM) had undergone total abdominal hysterectomy and bilateral salpingo-oophorectomy for benign gynecological diseases, such as uterine fibroids, ovarian masses, and resistant abnormal uterine bleeding. Women with natural menopause (NM) had intact uterus and ovaries.

The exclusion criteria for participants included type 1 diabetes mellitus (DM), and drug-dependent type 2 diabetes mellitus, hypertension (HT), except for stage 1 essential HT, cardiovascular diseases, chronic obstructive pulmonary disease, neurological or psychiatric diseases, use of antipsychotic and antidepressant drugs, thyroid dysfunction, pathological obesity, previous surgery in the past year, presence of a malignant disease, pelvic organ prolapse or any surgery for prolapse, any type of incontinence, alcohol or any drug abuse affecting sexual life, and homosexuality.

The exclusion criteria for the patients' sexual partners included type 1 diabetes mellitus, and drug-dependent type 2 diabetes mellitus, hypertension (HT) except for stage 1 essential HT, cardiovascular diseases, chronic obstructive pulmonary disease, neurological or psychiatric diseases, use of antipsychotic and antidepressant drugs, thyroid dysfunction, pathological obesity, previous surgery in the past 2 years, previous surgery for any prostate disease, symptomatic benign prostatic hyperplasia, and any sexual dysfunction such as erectile dysfunction or premature ejaculation. The Modified Female Sexual Function Index (FSFI), developed by Rosen et al., *was used to compare the sexual performance of the participants* [8], *including coital frequency and a face-to-face survey of six questions with all study groups.*

15.1.3 Result

Women's sexual performance can be influenced by many factors, *including age, parity, body mass index, marital status, sexual activity, menopausal status, residence, occupation, socio-economic level, education level, previous sexual trauma, and genitourinary surgeries, psychological factors, and sexual attitude, which is influenced by religion and beliefs, as well as the socio-demographic characteristics of the partner, such as age, body mass index, occupation, and education level* [9]. In the evaluation of sexual performance, some scoring indices have been developed with questions regarding hypoactive sexual desire disorder, frequency and satisfaction of intercourse, sexual arousal, orgasm, vaginal lubrication, and dyspareunia [8].

Using the *Golombok-Rust Inventory of Sexual Satisfaction*, Topatan et al. [10] reported a positive relationship between the intensity of surgical menopause symptoms and sexual dysfunction.

On this topic, Tucker et al. and Vermeulen et al. [11, 12] have found that premenopausal women undergoing salpingo-oophorectomy for risk reduction experienced greater sexual discomfort and greater dissatisfaction with their sexual life.

Scientific research has also asked the question: does surgical menopause affect female sexual performance differently than natural menopause?

In particular, the study by Kocku A. et al. [13] included 121 *women who had undergone surgical menopause, 122 women who had undergone natural menopause*, and all women had similar economic, sociocultural, and personal demographic profiles. They *were in postmenopause for at least 1 year and aged between 45 and 65 years*. The women were asked to complete a six-question survey on sexual performance parameters, including sexual desire, coital frequency, arousal, orgasm frequency, dyspareunia, and vaginal lubrication. These sexual performance parameters were compared between the surgical and natural menopause groups.

Except for vaginal lubrication, sexual performance parameters were not statistically different between the two groups. Vaginal lubrication in the surgical menopause group was lower compared to the natural menopause group. Serum levels of dehydroepiandrosterone sulfate, prolactin, and thyrotropin were not statistically different between the groups, while serum levels of estradiol and total testosterone in the surgical menopause group were lower than those in the natural menopause group.

In conclusion, women undergoing hysterectomy must overcome problems related to sexual and reproductive health. They often suffer from a drop in self-esteem due to sexual dysfunction and the inability to give birth, along with issues related to their recovery quality. The study by Afiyah RK et al. [14] described the relationships between recovery time and components of quality of life after hysterectomy. They recruited 103 women undergoing hysterectomy from various integrated health centers in the Surabaya community. ***The results show that there is a relationship between the recovery period and sexual activity***. However, there is no significant relationship between personal relationships during the recovery period and social support. *It follows that doctors and sex therapists should improve psychosocial support for women and families during recovery to avoid pathological stress and improve quality of life.*

15.2 Quality of Life in Men and Women After a Cancer Experience

Over 60% of people treated for cancer suffer from sexual dysfunction and hypoactive sexual desire disorder (HSDD) in the long term. However, less than 25% of those who have sexual problems receive help from a health professional. Although cancer-related sexual problems usually start with physiological damage due to cancer treatment, *the patient's adaptive abilities and the quality of the sexual relationship are crucial in sexual rehabilitation.* Obstacles to care for people treated for cancer include the lack of discussion with the oncology team and the reluctance to include a sex therapist in the therapeutic team. In repeated surveys, fewer than half of patients remember discussing sex or fertility with their healthcare providers, even during informed consent. *Practical guidelines on sexuality and cancer were published in 2017 by the American Society for Clinical Oncology (ASCO) and the National Comprehensive Cancer Network (NCCN).* Both agree: the oncology team should initiate discussions on sexuality and cancer during treatment planning and during follow-up visits. Psychosocial and medical evaluation should take place when a problem or concern is identified. It is; therefore, appropriate to propose multidisciplinary treatments, as sexual problems often have both psychological and physiological causes [15].

The adaptation of the guideline *Cancer Care Ontario (CCO) interventions to address sexual problems in people with cancer* provides recommendations for managing the adverse effects of sexual function that occur following the diagnosis and/or treatment of cancer.

The ASCO staff reviewed the guideline for evolutionary rigor and updated the bibliographic research. An ASCO expert group was formed to review the content and recommendations of the guideline.

The ASCO expert group determined that the recommendations of the 2016 CCO guideline are clear, comprehensive, and based on the most relevant scientific evidence. ASCO statements and modifications were added to adapt the CCO guideline to a wider audience [16].

It is recommended that there be a discussion with the patient, initiated by a member of the healthcare team, about the health and sexual dysfunction resulting from cancer or its treatment.

Psychosexual counseling should be offered to all cancer patients, with the aim of improving sexual response, body image, intimacy and relationship issues, and overall sexual functioning and satisfaction.

In women with symptoms of vaginal and/or vulvar atrophy, lubricants in addition to vaginal moisturizers can be tried as the first option. In some cases, low-dose vaginal estrogens, lidocaine, and dehydroepiandrosterone may also be considered. In men, drugs such as type 5 phosphodiesterase inhibitors can be useful and surgery remains an option for those who present symptoms or complications of treatment refractory to medical management. *Both women and men who exhibit vasomotor symptoms should be offered interventions for symptomatic improvement, including behavioral options such as cognitive behavioral therapy, slow breathing, and hypnosis, and medications such as venlafaxine and gabapentin.* Further information is available at: www.asco.org/survivorship-guidelines ***and*** www.asco.org/guidelineswiki.

In addition to this one study [17], a multidisciplinary specialist committee, as part of a broader *International Consultation*, worked with urological and sexual medicine societies for a period of 2 years to examine the outcome of chronic disease management on sexual function and satisfaction. The objectives, goals, data collection techniques, and report format were defined by a central committee. The scientific literature was reviewed, and it was confirmed that the data on the likelihood of specific sexual problems occurring with cancer and *its management vary depending on prediagnosis function, patient response, treatment team support, specific treatments used, proactive counseling, and efforts to mitigate potential problems.*

However, there are few published guidelines for managing sexual dysfunctions in men and women, despite the prevalence of these problems and the lack of attention they receive. Sexual function disorders in men include erectile dysfunction, hypoactive sexual desire disorder (HSDD), orgasm and ejaculation disorders, priapism, and Peyronie's disease.

An international consultation [18], in collaboration with the leading societies of urological and sexual medicine, brought together over 200 multidisciplinary experts from 60 countries in 17 consultation committees. The committee members established the scope and objectives for each chapter.

After an intense review of the data and available publications, the committees developed evidence-based guidelines in each area.

Recommendations and guidelines were developed for HSDD and male sexual dysfunction. These guidelines were developed as evidence-based, patient-centered, and with a multidisciplinary focus. For the clinical evaluation and diagnosis of ED, a basic evaluation was recommended for all patients, with optional and specialized tests reserved for special cases. A new treatment algorithm is proposed. This algorithm provides a clinically relevant guideline for the management of ED in the vast majority of men. New guidelines and treatment algorithms are provided for male orgasm and ejaculation disorders, including premature ejaculation, retrograde ejaculation, and delayed ejaculation. Finally, expert opinion-based guidelines are provided for the clinical management of priapism and Peyronie's disease.

Broadening the clinical observation, patients suffering from rectal cancer (RC) experience unique sources of discomfort, including sexual dysfunction and body image concerns, which can also cause discomfort among partners. The preliminary study by Acquati C et al. [19] examined the patterns of psychological distress, HSDD, sexual functioning, sexual distress, and relationship satisfaction among RC patient-partner couples at critical times during cancer treatment.

Twenty couples participated. ***Patients and partners completed a series of validated measures of psychological distress (ET), sexual functioning (FSFI; IIEF), sexual distress (GMSEX; Sexual Distress Scale), and relationship satisfaction (GMREL) at the time of diagnosis, 3 weeks after radiotherapy, 4 weeks after surgery, and after chemotherapy and surgery for ostomy closure***.

Relationship satisfaction remained high over time.

In this sample, 55% of patients and 78.9% of partners reported clinically significant rates of psychological distress at diagnosis, which dropped to 23% and 46% at the last evaluation. Satisfaction and sexual distress worsened for patients and partners between the start and the surgical procedure for the closure of the stoma. ***Both male and female participants reported statistically significant declines in sexual desire and sexual function from the beginning to the end of treatment***.

Regarding relationship satisfaction, psychological health, and sexual health outcomes seem more vulnerable to the effects of rectal cancer treatment during the first year after diagnosis, for both patients and partners, and for both men and women.

A total of 394 (66.2% women) oncology patients treated curatively were recruited, with 34% of patients in treatment and 66% of patients in follow-up after primary treatment (out of treatment group), who completed *the EORTC QLQ-SH22 and the EORTC QLQ-C30*, assessing SH and quality of life [20].

Compared to patients out of treatment, patients in active cancer treatment experienced lower sexual satisfaction, HSDD, and higher levels of fatigue. The effects of treatment on sexual activity decreased with the completion of treatment.

Patients undergoing intensified treatment—chemotherapy, radiotherapy or endocrine treatment) reported more treatment effects (subscale EORTC QLQ-SH22) compared to patients undergoing only surgical intervention.

Despite available support, sexual needs are the most frequently reported unmet need **among men with prostate cancer**, which could be due to low rates of help-seeking. Using the Ecological Systems Framework as a theoretical foundation, we conducted a scoping review of the available literature to understand which factors influence help-seeking behavior for sexual problems after prostate cancer treatment among men who had received treatment [21].

Following PRISMA guidelines, a systematic search was conducted on *Medline, PsychInfo, Embase, Emcare* and *Scopus* to identify studies on adult patients with post-treatment prostate cancer, reporting barriers and/or facilitators to seeking help for sexual health problems. Quality assessments were conducted using the Joanna Briggs Institute evaluation tools and the results were summarized qualitatively. **Of the 3870 unique results, only 30 studies met the inclusion criteria**. In general, the studies were considered of moderate to good quality, although only six used standardized measures to assess help-seeking behavior. Barriers and facilitators for seeking sexual help were identified at all five levels of the Ecological Systems Framework, including *age, type of treatment and previous experience of help-seeking (individual level), communication with health professionals and partner support (microsystem), financial cost and accessibility of support (meso/exosystem) and finally embarrassment, masculinity, cultural norms, and sexual minority (macrosystem).*

15.3 A Thorough Review by the Disciplinary Committee of Adolescent and Young Adult Oncology of the Children's Oncology Group

Sexual function is a fundamental aspect of quality of life among adolescent and young adult (AYA) survivors of cancer, ages 15–39 years. Sexual function includes physical, psychosocial and developmental factors that contribute to sexual health, all negatively influenced by cancer and treatment. However, limited information is available to inform the care of AYA cancer survivors in this regard.

The review [22], conducted by the ***Children's Oncology Group AYA Oncology Discipline Committee***, summarizes the available literature on sexual function among AYA cancer survivors, including relevant psychosexual aspects of romantic relationships and body image. The findings suggest that, overall; AYA cancer survivors experience a significant burden of sexual dysfunction. Both physical and psychosocial sequelae affect the sexual health of young patients.

Interventions are needed to support sexual health and psychosexual adaptation after cancer treatment. Collaboration is necessary between the ***Children's Oncology Group and adult-focused cooperative groups within the National Clinical Trials Network of the National Cancer Institute*** to promote the prospective evaluation of sexual dysfunction, hypoactive sexual desire disorder (HSDD), and to test interventions aimed at improving sexual health among AYA oncology patients. For many adolescents and young adults (AYA) affected by cancer, psychosexual well-being is compromised due to the onset of the disease during a vulnerable phase of sexual development. So far, previous studies have focused on the psychosexual well-being of adult patients, largely ignoring AYAs. Moreover, the few studies that have investigated the psychosexual well-being of AYAs have been prematurely quantitative in nature, limited by the lack of an in-depth exploration of the unique psychosexual experiences of AYA survivors.

The study by Dobinson KA et al. [23], conducted semi-structured interviews with 11 AYA patients aged between 15 and 45 at the time of diagnosis. The analysis of constant comparison data gave rise to the *Pathways to Problems* model, which denotes the paths to unmet psychosexual needs among AYA patients. Participants experienced an identity conflict, in which there was an incongruity between their chronological age and their self-perceived age. The experience of identity conflict, combined with changes in intimate relationships, changes in priorities, physician assumptions, and inadequate support, contributed to the onset of unmet psychosexual needs. Six areas of unmet psychosexual needs were identified: fertility issues, sexual communication, HSDD, management of side effects, dating and disclosure, relationship with other AYAs, and reconciliation of identity conflict.

The study by Aldiwan A et al. [24] includes interviews with eight AYAs diagnosed with testicular cancer (TCS). The results were analyzed using interpretative phenomenological analysis. The questions explored experiences related to diagnosis and treatment, how they influenced the development of their psychosexual identity (sexual relationships and self-image), and the meanings attributed to the experiences. From the data, four group experiential themes were developed: "Dealing with the Shock," "Fear and Weight of Responsibility," "The People Closest to Me," and "Sense of Change" in relationships with family and friends.

AYA TCS experiences can lead to the adoption of traditional male traits (stoicism) or the abandonment of traditionally male traits (violence and aggressiveness). AYA TCS also described feelings of insecurity compared to other men. Psychosexual input could help manage stoicism and feelings of inferiority compared to men with two testicles.

Comparing the study by Wong AWK et al. [25] reveals the phenomenological experiences of AYA survivors based on their language. A total of 1993 AYA oncology patients (post-treatment) were recruited and included in 58 studies (78% individual interviews). The average age was 27.6 years with an average of 8.6 years after primary treatment, across a heterogeneous group of cancer diagnoses.

Thirteen themes were identified, including symptoms, HSDD, sexual function, reproductive health, emotional well-being, health management, healthcare system, social interaction, romantic relationships, cancer disclosure, normality, career development and occupation, and school and financial concerns. Additionally, 48 sub-themes covering areas such as fertility, integrative health services, cancer disclosure counseling, family interaction, and insurance challenges were identified.

In particular, insurance and job issues are two themes of young Asians that are underdeveloped in the literature. One study [26] recruited 23 AYA oncology patients and 18 healthcare providers (HCP) who cared for AYA oncology patients, structured 11 focus group sessions. A thematic content analysis was conducted to identify the main themes that emerged. Similar themes emerged from the AYA and HCP focus groups. Most AYA patients were anxious to return to work after treatment. However, some young people were worried about not meeting expectations and had difficulty disclosing their clinical history. Conversely, several AYA patients leveraged their cancer experience to strengthen job opportunities. Despite challenges due to cancer complications and work restrictions, AYA patients preferred to be treated normally. Young AYAs also expressed concerns about the inadequate insurance coverage and lack of information on this topic.

Contrary to expectations, Asian AYA patients are motivated to return to work and face work-related challenges. Inadequate insurance coverage remains an urgent concern despite the availability of public health insurance and subsidies. The study also suggests that "career coaches and financial advisors" should be incorporated into survivor care to assist AYA survivors.

15.4 Conclusions

Although international guidelines and scientific literature strongly recommend the presence of a psychosexual therapist in the oncology team, even today few Institutes consider this role as fundamental for the sexual recovery of individuals and couples. The psychosexual therapist, in my clinical experience, should be present from the delivery of the histological report. Observing the emotional reactions of the patient would make it possible from the outset to predict therapeutic compliance during surgical or oncological treatments. Oncology patients disregard a lot of information: after an oncological diagnosis, they enter into post-traumatic stress that deepens following the preoperative surgery or oncological treatments. What does this mean? These patients, for 90–120 days, undergo neurological and psychological changes dependent on the recommended treatment. This means mood disorder, HSDD, inadequacy, loneliness, depression, alterations in sleep quality, chronic fatigue, and gastrointestinal alterations. And the partners? They often feel neglected, and out of fear of losing thc patient, they only think about survival. "Sexuality doesn't matter; he or she needs to heal," is the expression most often stated by partners, while the patient silently feels that their femininity or virility has been set aside, and they will no longer be the same individual as before. If the psychosexual therapist shared these neuro-vegetative and psychological changes in advance, surely, the patient, adult or adolescent, would feel part of a team that supports them and believes in their femininity or virility, not least by educating the partner or the family to respect the psychological needs and social role of the patient [27].

References

1. Luo F, Link M, Grabenhorst C, Lynn B. Low sexual desire in breast cancer survivors and patients: a review. Sex Med Rev. 2022;10(3):367–75.
2. Hummel SB, Hahn DEE, van Lankveld JJDM, Oldenburg HSA, Broomans E, Aaronson NK. Factors associated with specific diagnostic and statistical manual of mental disorders, fourth edition sexual dysfunctions in breast cancer survivors: a study of patients and their partners. J Sex Med. 2017;14(10):1248–59.

3. Tucker PE, Saunders C, Bulsara MK, Tan JJ, Salfinger SG, Green H, Cohen PA. Sexuality and quality of life in women with a prior diagnosis of breast cancer after risk-reducing salpingo-oophorectomy. Breast. 2016;30:26–31.
4. El-Toukhy TA, Hefni MA, Davies AE, Mahadevan S. The effect of different types of hysterectomy on urinary and sexual functions: a prospective study. J Obstet Gynaecol. 2004;24(4):420–5.
5. Aziz A, Bergquist C, Nordholm L, et al. Prophylactic ovariectomy during elective hysterectomy: effects on psychological well-being at one year follow-up and its correlations with sexuality. Maturitas. 2005;51(4):349–57.
6. Tucker PE, Cohen PA. Review article: sexuality and risk-reducing salpingo-oophorectomy. Int J Gynecol Cancer. 2017;27(4):847–52.
7. Bıldırcın FD, Özdeş EK, Karlı P, Özdemir AZ, Kökçü A. Does type of menopause affect the sex lives of women? Med Sci Monit. 2020;26:e921811.
8. Rosen C, Brown J, Heiman S, et al. The female sexual function index (FSFI): a multidimensional self-assessment tool for the evaluation of female sexual function. J Sex Marital Ther. 2000;26(2):191–208.
9. Moghasemi S, Ozgoli G, Ahmadi F, Simbar M. Sexual experience of Iranian women in middle age: a qualitative approach. Int J Commun Based Nurs Midwifery. 2018;6(1):47–55.
10. Topatan S, Yıldız H. Symptoms experienced by women entering natural and surgical menopause and their relationship with sexual functions. Health Care Women Int. 2012;33(6):525–39.
11. Vermeulen RFM, Beurden MV, Korse CM, Kenter GG. Impact of risk-reducing salpingo-oophorectomy in premenopausal women. Climacteric. 2017;20(3):212–21.
12. Tucker PE, Bulsara MK, Salfinger SG, et al. The effects of preoperative menopausal status and hormone replacement therapy (HRT) on sexuality and quality of life after risk-reducing salpingo-oophorectomy. Maturitas. 2016;85:42–8.
13. Kokcu A, Kurtoglu E, Bildircin D, Celik H, Kaya A, Alper T. Does surgical menopause affect sexual performance differently from natural menopause? J Sex Med. 2015 Jun;12(6):1407–14.
14. Afiyah RK, Wahyuni CU, Prasetyo B, Dwi Winarno D. Recovery time period and quality of life after hysterectomy. J Public Health Res. 2020;9(2):1837.
15. Schover LR. Sexual quality of life in men and women after cancer. Climacteric. 2019;22(6):553–7.
16. Carter J, Lacchetti C, Andersen BL, Barton DL, Bolte S, Damast S, Diefenbach MA, DuHamel K, Florendo J, Ganz PA, Goldfarb S, Hallmeyer S, Kushner DM, Rowland JH. Interventions to address sexual problems in people with cancer: American Society of Clinical Oncology clinical practice guideline adaptation of Cancer Care Ontario guideline. J Clin Oncol. 2018;36(5):492–511. https://doi.org/10.1200/JCO.2017.75.8995. Epub 2017 Dec 11.
17. Sadovsky R, Basson R, Krychman M, Morales AM, Schover L, Wang R, Incrocci L. Cancer and sexual problems. J Sex Med. 2010;7(1 Pt 2):349–73.
18. Lue TF, Giuliano F, Montorsi F, Rosen RC, Andersson KE, Althof S, Christ G, Hatzichristou D, Hirsch M, Kimoto Y, Lewis R, McKenna K, MacMahon C, Morales A, Mulcahy J, Padma-Nathan H, Pryor J, de Tejada IS, Shabsigh R, Wagner G. Summary of the recommendations on sexual dysfunctions in men. J Sex Med. 2004;1(1):6–23.
19. Acquati C, Hendren S, Wittmann D, Reese JB, Karam E, Duby A, Dunn KB, Kayser K. Psychological and sexual distress in rectal cancer patients and partners. Psychooncology. 2022;31(6):920–8.
20. Oberguggenberger AS, Engele VI, Schmalz C, Nordin A, Bjelic-Radisic V, Lanceley A, Kuljanic K, Jensen PT, Frøding LP, Creutzberg CL, Zimmermann K, Serpentini S, Arraras JI, Nagele E, Toelen H, Greimel E, EORTC Quality of Life Group. The impact of curative cancer treatment on sexual health – clinical results from the EORTC QLQ-SH22 validation study. BMC Cancer. 2024;24(1):1374. https://doi.org/10.1186/s12885-024-13123-7. PMID: 39523323; PMCID: PMC11552421.
21. Charlick M, Tiruye T, Ettridge K, O'Callaghan M, Sara S, Jay A, Beckmann K. Prostate cancer related sexual dysfunction and barriers to help seeking: a scoping review. Psychooncology. 2024;33(8):e9303. https://doi.org/10.1002/pon.9303.

22. Cherven B, Sampson A, Bober SL, Bingen K, Frederick N, Freyer DR, Quinn GP. Sexual health among adolescent and young adult cancer survivors: a scoping review from the children's oncology group adolescent and young adult oncology discipline committee. CA Cancer J Clin. 2021;71(3):250–63. https://doi.org/10.3322/caac.21655. Epub 2020 Dec 7. PMID: 33283888; PMCID: PMC8678924.
23. Dobinson KA, Hoyt MA, Seidler ZE, Beaumont AL, Hullmann SE, Lawsin CR. A grounded theory investigation into the psychosexual unmet needs of adolescent and young adult cancer survivors. J Adolesc Young Adult Oncol. 2016;5(2):135–45.
24. Aldiwan A, McParland J, Leeuwerik T, Stoneham S, Williamson M, Christie D. An interpretative phenomenological analysis of the psychosexual identity development in adolescent and young adult survivors of testicular cancer. Clin Child Psychol Psychiatry. 2024;29(4):1432–47.
25. Wong AWK, Chang TT, Christopher K, Lau SCL, Beaupin LK, Love B, Lipsey KL, Feuerstein M. Patterns of unmet needs in adolescent and young adult (AYA) cancer survivors: in their own words. J Cancer Surviv. 2017;11(6):751–64.
26. Tan CJ, Ke Y, Ng T, Tan IMJ, Goh WL, Poon E, Farid M, Neo PSH, Srilatha B, Chan A. Work- and insurance-related issues among Asian adolescent and young-adult cancer survivors: a qualitative study. Support Care Cancer. 2020;28(12):5901–9.
27. Longhi EV, Franco G, Colombo F. Psychosexual counseling in andrological surgery. Springer; 2000.

HSDD and Multiple Sclerosis

16

Abstract

Multiple sclerosis (MS) is the most common disabling condition among young adults, with a myriad of potential effects on neurological function, including sensory and autonomic functions (Kingwell et al. BMC Neurol 13(1):1–13, 2013). MS can also affect sexual function indirectly through other physical disabilities, such as spasticity or bladder dysfunction; as a side effect of medications; and through psychosocial mechanisms, such as the presence of depression (Foley et al. Mult Scler 19(9):1197–203, 2013). A disturbed sexual function can have particularly harmful effects on couple relationships and on the quality of life related to mental health, as is well demonstrated in a large sample of the *North American Research Committee on Multiple Sclerosis (NARCOMS) Registry of 6,183 PwMS* (Schairer et al. Mult Scler 20(5):610–6, 2014).

Keywords

Multiple sclerosis, Sexual function, Sexual dysfunction, Epidemiology, Prevalence, Quality of life · Depression · Disability · Multiple sclerosis · Urodynamic function · Quality of life · Urodynamic function

16.1 Introduction

A review of seven studies from 1995, with a total of 455 women and 326 men with *multiple sclerosis*, highlighted a percentage of 33–75% for women and 47–75% for men of confirmed diagnoses [4]. This review has often been cited in subsequent articles as a prevalence of 40–80% for women and 50–90% for men [5]. A more precise prevalence of SD is difficult to determine because definitions are sometimes inconsistent.

According to the World Health Organization (WHO), SD is a syndrome that includes one or more of the following: **lack or loss of sexual desire, sexual**

E. V. Longhi, *Hypoactive Sexual Desire Disorder*,
https://doi.org/10.1007/978-3-032-00659-2_16

aversion, and lack of sexual enjoyment; failure of genital response (erectile dysfunction in men and vaginal dryness or lack of lubrication in women); **orgasmic dysfunction; premature ejaculation, vaginismus, and dyspareunia** [6].

Primary SD refers to the direct impairment of sexual responses or feelings through neurological damage in the central nervous system. This can lead to symptoms such as HSDD, erectile dysfunction, anorgasmia, and decreased sensitivity. **Secondary SD** occurs when physical changes indirectly affect sexual responses, not related to specific nerve pathways to the genitals, including fatigue, muscle stiffness, spasticity or weakness, and bladder or bowel dysfunction. **Tertiary SD** refers to psychosocial problems associated with body image, emotional challenges, and cultural influences, including the commonly experienced effects of depression on sexual function and low self-esteem that indirectly affect sexual function [7]. Several studies have identified demographic variables associated with sexual dysfunction, including age, number of children, education, and duration of the relationship, while disease characteristics such as the level of disability, duration, and type of multiple sclerosis also play a role.

The study by Tepavcevic DK et al. [8] estimated the frequency, type, and intensity of sexual dysfunction in patients with multiple sclerosis, and investigated its influence on all domains of quality of life. A sample of 109 patients with multiple sclerosis was recruited. Sexual dysfunction was quantified using the Szasz Sexual Functioning Scale. Health-related quality of life was measured by a disease-specific instrument, MSQoL-54.

The presence of at least one symptom of SD was found in about 84% of men and 85% of women. The main complaints in women were: *HSDD, difficulty achieving orgasm, and decreased vaginal lubrication*, in men, the main complaints were *reduced libido, incomplete erections, and premature ejaculation.*

In women, statistically significant negative correlations were observed between the presence and level of SD and the domains of quality of life for all subscales, except for the pain subscale.

In men, negative correlations were also observed for all domains but were statistically significant for physical health, physical role limitations, social function, health discomfort, sexual function, and satisfaction with sexual function.

16.2 Psychosexual Aspects

The study by Marck CH et al. [9] evaluated the prevalence of SD and satisfaction with sexual function in an international sample of people with multiple sclerosis (PwMS), recruited online as part of the ***Health Outcomes and Lifestyle in a Sample of People with Multiple Sclerosis (HOLISM) study***. The following were also evaluated: the associations between disease characteristics, fatigue, risk of depression, and demographic data with sexual function and satisfaction, as well as lifestyle.

Participants were recruited through online platforms, including social media, websites, and forums involving people with multiple sclerosis, most of which focused on health and lifestyle.

The web-based tool SurveyMonkey was used to provide respondents with a participant information sheet, an electronic consent indicator, and the survey itself. The inclusion criteria were adults aged 18 years or older who self-reported a formal diagnosis of *multiple sclerosis* by a physician. Since the survey was in English, only English-speaking participants were included [10].

The online survey took about 40 minutes to complete.

The sexual function scale and the quality of life satisfaction item in Multiple Sclerosis Quality of Life-54 (MSQOL-54) were used. The sexual function scale covered: hypoactive sexual desire disorder, erection difficulties (for men), lubrication difficulties (for women), difficulty achieving orgasm, and ability to satisfy a sexual partner.

These items had four options (and corresponding score): "not a problem" (100), "a small problem" (66.6), "a modest problem" (33.3) and "a big problem" (0).

In addition, satisfaction was assessed with a single item: "Overall, how satisfied are you with your sexual function in the last 4 weeks?" The corresponding responses were "satisfied" (including "very satisfied" and "quite satisfied") and "not satisfied" (including "neither satisfied nor dissatisfied," "quite dissatisfied" and "very dissatisfied").

Of the 2,469 respondents with confirmed multiple sclerosis, a total of 2,062 completed the items on sexual function.

Overall, 54.5% were classified as having sexual dysfunction, (49.7% of men and 55.6% of women).

Lack of sexual interest was identified as a serious problem for 39.6%, including 29.8% of men and 41.8% of women.

Following: difficulty with erection or lubrication (40.7% of men and 30.9% of women); inability or difficulty in achieving an orgasm (30.1% of men and 36.0% of women); fatigue of satisfying (28.9% of men and 19.7% of women). Patients with sexual dysfunction were less likely to be satisfied compared to the control group.

The fact remains that sexual function is often not a standard part of the consultation with healthcare professionals for people with multiple sclerosis (PwMS) [11], despite requests for inclusion [12], and is therefore often underdiagnosed [13].

Among the factors conditioning sexual function, HSDD, *depression, and fatigue* [14] *play a significant role.*

Studies on sexual dysfunction in patients with *multiple sclerosis* report a wide range: between 40% and 80% in women and 50% and 90% in men [14]. Almost half (47%) of American women [15] and 61% of Israeli women [16] suffered from hypoactive sexual desire disorder and sexual dysfunction, while in Turkey, most women (75–80.1%) reported sexual dysfunction [17, 18].

In addition, patients with MS show less energy compared to healthy people, and their energy is particularly depleted in the afternoon and at night, increasing the likelihood that they may avoid sexual activity. This is why patients with MS are often advised to engage in sexual activity in the morning to reduce the incidence of sexual problems caused by fatigue [19].

In another study by McCabe MP et al. (20), *how the sexuality and relationships of people with multiple sclerosis (MS) differ from those of the general population was examined.*

The study involved 381 patients, including 144 men and 237 women, with MS and 291 from the control group, including 101 men and 190 women.

Sexual satisfaction, sexual dysfunction, relational satisfaction, and coping style were evaluated among all respondents. Information was also obtained from people with multiple sclerosis (MS) regarding the age of onset and diagnosis of symptoms, as well as the severity of symptoms.

Overall, men with multiple sclerosis (MS) experienced a higher frequency of sexual dysfunction and hypoactive sexual desire disorder (HSDD) compared to men in the general population, while women with multiple sclerosis (MS) differed from women of the general population only in their levels of masturbation and numbness in the genital area.

Coping strategies and levels of cognitive functioning were important predictors of sexual satisfaction, sexual dysfunction, and relationship satisfaction for women with multiple sclerosis, but fewer coping or health-related factors predicted these variables among men with multiple sclerosis. *The results of this study highlight factors related to sexual satisfaction and interpersonal relationships.*

16.3 How Do These Relationships Change Over Time?

A longitudinal investigation was also conducted on the impact of coping style and disease-related variables among people with multiple sclerosis and the general population on sexual and relational functioning [21].

Both men (120) and women (201) with multiple sclerosis and men (79) and women (160) from the general population participated in the study at two different times, 6 months apart. *People with multiple sclerosis experienced lower levels of sexual activity, sexual satisfaction, and relationship satisfaction, and higher levels of sexual dysfunction.*

For respondents who had been diagnosed with MS for less than 7 years, levels of sexual activity in the past 6 months appeared to be decrease for HSDD and for frequency of sexual intercourse.

After 2 years the follow-up appears illustrative.

A 2-year follow-up study of 99 patients with diagnosed multiple sclerosis collected information on sexual and sphincter disorders through face-to-face structured interviews [22]. Disability, independence, cognitive performance, and psychological functioning were also evaluated. Spearman rank correlation analyses, corrected for multiple comparisons, and linear regression analyses were performed to test the relationship between variables and remove the effect of potential confounding covariates.

The percentage of patients with sexual dysfunction remained over 70% and did not change during the 2-year follow-up, but the extent and number of symptoms significantly increased. Significantly, more patients than before the study had resorted to counseling and discussed sexual issues with doctors.

In the univariate analysis, changes in sexual function over time were correlated with changes in bladder function and EDSS score, but the multivariate analysis showed that only bladder dysfunction was independently correlated with sexual dysfunction and HSDD.

According to a recent study by Schairer et al. [23], sexual dysfunction can potentially have a more significant impact on mental health and quality of life (QoL), compared with the sum of neurological and functional deficits in patients.

The lack of training and knowledge among professionals regarding sexuality in people with MS could be resolved by educating health professionals on the management and evaluation of sexuality in these patients [24]. Therefore, for this to happen, questionnaires for the measurement of sexual function that have been validated in people with MS must be available. The only reliable, valid tools for assessing sexuality, including all possible causes of dysfunction in both men and women with MS, are the *Multiple Sclerosis Intimacy and Sexuality Questionnaire-19* (MSISQ-19) and its shortened version, the *Multiple Sclerosis Intimacy and Sexuality Questionnaire-15* (MSISQ-15) [25].

This questionnaire consists of three subscales that cover most of the causes of sexual dysfunction in people with MS: primary causes related to the involvement of the central nervous system, secondary causes related to the physical aspects of the disease or resulting from its treatment, and tertiary causes resulting from sociocultural and psycho-emotional factors [26].

In the study by Carrillo et al. [27], sexual dysfunctions were evaluated according to the time of onset of the pathological course; ***the prevalence ranges between 50% and 90% and can be secondary to demyelinating lesions in the spinal cord and/or brain or caused by symptoms that do not directly involve the nervous system*** (fatigue; psychological, social and cultural factors; etc.). Although its prevalence and impact on quality of life are well known, sexual dysfunction is still often underestimated.

Five questionnaires were evaluated that could identify the presence of sexual dysfunction in patients with multiple sclerosis (MS) and determine its etiology, aiding in the decision-making process for treatment. MS should be understood as a complex disease that includes and compromises various aspects of patients' health and goes beyond the simple measurement of disability.

Furthermore: the study by Kaplan TB et al. [28] investigated whether there were gender differences and sexual dysfunctions between men and women diagnosed with MS. The analysis includes *person with MS enrolled in the Comprehensive Longitudinal Investigation of Multiple Sclerosis at the Brigham and Women's Hospital (CLIMB), who completed*: ***Multiple Sclerosis Quality of Life-54 (MSQOL-54), Modified Fatigue Impact Scale (MFIS), and Center for Epidemiologic Studies Depression Scale (CES-D).***

The results were stratified by sex. Seven hundred two persons with MS (526 females, 176 males, average age 42.2) were included in the cross-sectional analysis. Data from 341 persons with MS were used in the 3-year longitudinal analysis.

Increases in age, disease duration, and disability were associated with a reduction in function, sexual satisfaction, and hypoactive sexual desire disorder (HSDD) to the same extent in males and females.

Age and disease duration were associated with reduced function and sexual satisfaction in males and females. In females, function was significantly associated with disability. Males had stronger associations with sexual function in domains related to emotional well-being, health perception, and overall quality of life. Males had more evident associations with emotional, social satisfaction, and physical health.

16.4 Underdiagnosed MS Traits and Couple Relationships

The fact that sexual function (SD) remains underdiagnosed can be explained by some ***barriers reported by both neurologists and patients***. The main barriers to the evaluation of SD found in one 2022 survey [29] were *lack of time, lack of knowledge, or the presence of a companion during the consultation*. Previous studies have identified similar barriers perceived by healthcare providers (HCP), such as lack of time, *lack of knowledge, and the presence of a companion during the consultation* [24].

Moreover, HCPs are concerned because they are not sure that patients want to be asked about sexual function and some HCPs think that this topic can be invasive [30]. In fact, most patients perceive the need to talk about their sexual function.

Furthermore, neurologists usually explore SD using informal questions; however, more than half understand that there are questionnaires on sexual dysfunction for MS. *This behavior can be explained by the lack of available time during the consultation or the lack of training on how to apply and interpret these questionnaires.*

Although most Colombian neurologists ask for information about SD, only 13% initiate treatment, and most of them refer the patient to another specialist. This is in line with previous studies that reported that satisfaction with SD treatment was generally poor [31].

Similarly, Redelman reported that more than half of patients with SD did not get help for their problem (33). This reflects the fact that it is not only important to ask and diagnose but also to treat SD in these patients.

Attempts to overcome these limitations have also been made in Italy. The study by Carotenuto A. et al. [33] aimed to validate the ***Multiple Sclerosis Intimacy and Sexuality Questionnaire (MSISQ-19)*** for Italian patients with MS. Test-retest stability and concurrent internal and external validity were examined by Pearson correlation coefficients.

A total of **369** MS patients (323 women and 46 men) were enrolled.

The Italian *MSISQ-19* showed a Cronbach's alpha of 0.92. The total scores of the test and retest of the MSISQ-19 were correlated ($r = 0.48$, $p = 0.01$). The total score of the *MSISQ-19* was also correlated with the primary, secondary, and tertiary subscales ($p < 0.001$). The Italian version of the *MSISQ-19* showed satisfactory internal consistency and reliability with moderately adequate test-retest reproducibility, suggesting that it could be used as a valuable measure of sexual dysfunction in the Italian population.

The MSISQ-19 has also been translated into Turkish, Greek, Persian, and French versions.

A further limitation in sexuality and HSDD in patients with MS is "dysphagia" (difficulty swallowing).

Dysphagia is associated with significant morbidity and mortality, has a profound impact on quality of life, but is **underreported by patients**. One study [34] investigated the psychometric properties of the questionnaire Dysphagia in Multiple Sclerosis (DYMUS).

A total of 153 MS patients and 104 healthy patients for the control group completed the *DYMUS and the Eating Assessment Tool 10* (EAT-10).

The mod-DYMUS (comprised of items 1 and 3–7) demonstrated improved internal consistency (Cronbach's alpha 0.903) and inter-item correlation coefficients (0.558–0.657), good test-retest reliability, excellent criterion validity, and improved convergent validity. Patients had a significantly higher average mod-DYMUS score compared to patients in the control group ($P < 0.001$). Dysphagic patients (EAT-10 ≥ 3) had a significantly higher mod-DYMUS compared to non-dysphagic patients ($P < 0.001$). A strong and significant positive correlation was noted between the mod-DYMUS and the EAT-10 ($P < 0.001$). A mod-DYMUS score equal to or greater than 1 indicates dysphagia.

Overcoming reticence about the sexuality of people with multiple sclerosis (MS) patients requires remembering that MS affects not only the individuals with the disease but also their partners.

BUSCH AK et al. [35] explored the current level of knowledge about managing MS in couple relationships: studies were searched in the *CINAHL*, *Medline*, and *PsycINFO* databases using the following keywords: multiple sclerosis, spouses, couples, married couple, dyadic system, dyadic systems, and dyads. The results were interpreted in the context of the "*Evolutionary-Contextual Model of Couples Facing Chronic Illness over the Course of Adult Life*".

The results clearly showed that both partners experience feelings such as uncertainty, fear, depression, and distress. Coping in a relationship with the often-changing situations of the disease and the associated stress is better in couples who constantly exchange perceptions and confront mental and physical tensions.

However, although some positive aspects of managing MS as a couple were identified, MS has been associated with higher rates of relationship breakdown and a worse quality of life (QoL) for both people in the relationship—especially if the person with MS experiences a decline in mental or physical health or develops disabilities. Modifying lifestyle-related risk factors has been associated with better outcomes for people with MS, including physical and mental health—related QoL, and these improved outcomes can lead to better experiences for their partners.

Studies [36] have explored the perspectives and experiences of partners of people with MS when those individuals participated in an intensive residential workshop on healthy lifestyle to understand the impact of MS and lifestyle modification on these partners' experiences in their relationship. Within the framework of Heidegger's interpretive phenomenology, semi-structured interviews were thematically analyzed. The participants were in a marital relationship with people with MS who had attended an intensive residential workshop on modifying lifestyle-related risk factors between 2002 and 2016. The participants lived in Australia, New Zealand, the United Kingdom, and Europe. Three main themes related to couple relationships were identified: providing support, remaining accomplices, and the strong bond. Aspects of these themes, not commonly reported previously, included the personal and relational benefits experienced by providing support with lifestyle modification, improved communication, and the resulting greater sense of closeness.

16.5 Conclusions

People with multiple sclerosis (PwMS) often experience uncertainty and fear for their future. The partners of PwMS can share their concerns and experience fears regarding their future, limitations in their lives, hypoactive sexual desire disorder (HSDD), and the decreased ability to work and become "a caregiver" [37].

For people with MS, modifying lifestyle-related risk factors has been associated with better health outcomes. For those who participated in residential lifestyle modification workshops (RLMWs), improved and lasting health outcomes have been demonstrated. Whether the improved outcomes for people with MS who engage in lifestyle modification translate into better perceptions of the future by the partners remains to be explored.

The perspectives of partners of people with MS who had participated in an RLMW and the impact that the disease and their commitment to lifestyle modification had on their partners' views of the future were explored. The analysis of 21 semi-structured interviews used a methodology inspired by Heidegger's interpretive phenomenology.

Three themes emerged: "uncertainty," "planning for the future," and "control, empowerment, and security." Subthemes included MS and lifestyle modification as catalysts for positive change; development of a sense of control and empowerment; and hope, optimism, and positivity. Lifestyle modification can bring benefits not only to people with MS but also to their partners and should be considered part of the traditional management of MS. However, this unpredictability can cause feelings of helplessness for the partner and a sense of inability to control their own future.

For partners in caregiving roles, the wide range of manifestations and the unpredictable progression of MS pose additional practical and psychological challenges.

Rollero C et al. [38] conducted a qualitative study following a grounded theory approach in this regard. Twenty-four men, husbands or partners of woman diagnosed with MS, were interviewed in depth. Five main themes emerged: caregiving as a full-time job; changes in the couple; the importance of social support and social life; gender specifics; and fear of the future [39].

Despite recent advances in treatment, many people with (MS) require ongoing care and support. Caregivers may experience a burden due to their role, with potential implications for quality of life (QOL).

The experience of those providing care for MS is highly variable and can be predicted by a variety of factors related to the care recipient, the provider, and the context. Emotional burden is not the only characteristic associated with caregiving; emerging research suggests a range of ways in which caregivers can be better supported.

A recent report [40] found that caring for people with MS can negatively impact the physical and mental health of the caregiver, as well as affect their financial situation and employment status.

Few countries collect statistics on the number of those providing care for MS patients [41]; however, a recent large-scale analysis with nearly 17,000 people with MS suggested that 46% received informal care from family members [42]. While this figure is broadly consistent with other estimates [43], some studies report that up to 58% of people with MS receive informal care [44] with care requirements increasing significantly with increasing levels of disability. Given an estimate of over 2.2 million cases of MS worldwide, we can therefore extrapolate that there are more than one million caregivers globally.

Currently, informal care for people with MS is most commonly provided by spouses, with recent estimates of spousal care ranging from 53% [45] to 70%.

In a study conducted in Mexico, female caregivers of people with MS reported dedicating nearly twice the time to caregiving compared to male caregivers (79 versus 48 hours a week) [46], and they had performed their caregiving role for nearly three times longer.

A recent study found that caregivers of people with MS had a lower health-related quality of life compared to non-caregivers [47], with 68% experiencing pathological anxiety and 44% experiencing pathological depression, using the Hospital Anxiety and Depression Scale (HADS). It was also found that MS caregivers experienced high levels of fatigue, depression, and anger [48]. This is in line with recent findings from other disease domains, where it has been reported that caregiving negatively impacts on the caregiver's health and quality of life [49].

References

1. Kingwell E, Marriott JJ, Jetté N, et al. Incidence and prevalence of multiple sclerosis in Europe: a systematic review. BMC Neurol. 2013;13(1):1–13. https://doi.org/10.1186/1471-2377-13-128.
2. Foley FW, Zemon V, Campagnolo D, et al. The questionnaire on intimacy and sexuality in multiple sclerosis: revalidation and development of a 15-item version with a large US sample. Mult Scler. 2013;19(9):1197–203.
3. Schairer LC, Foley FW, Zemon V, et al. The impact of sexual dysfunction on health-related quality of life in people with multiple sclerosis. Mult Scler. 2014;20(5):610–6.
4. Dupont S. Multiple sclerosis and sexual functioning - a review. Clin Rehabil. 1995;9(2):135–41.

5. Calabro RS, De Luca R, Conti-Nibali V, Reitano S, Leo A, Bramanti P. Sexual dysfunction in male patients with multiple sclerosis: the need for counseling! Int J Neurosci. 2014;124(8):547–57.
6. World Health Organization. International Statistical Classification of Diseases and Related Health Problems 10th Revision (ICD-10)-WHO Version for 2016. 2015; http://apps.who.int/classifications/icd10/browse/2016/en#!/F52.0.
7. Kessler TM, Fowler CJ, Panicker JN. Sexual dysfunction in multiple sclerosis. Expert Rev Neurother. 2009;9(3):341–50. https://doi.org/10.1586/14737175.9.3.341.
8. Tepavcevic DK, Kostic J, Basuroski ID, Stojsavljevic N, Pekmezovic T, Drulovic J. The impact of sexual dysfunction on the quality of life measured by MSQoL-54 in patients with multiple sclerosis. Mult Scler. 2008;14(8):1131–6. https://doi.org/10.1177/1352458508093619. Epub 2008 Jul 16.
9. Marck CH, Jelinek PL, Weiland TJ, Hocking JS, De Livera AM, Taylor KL, Neate SL, Pereira NG, Jelinek GA. Sexual function in multiple sclerosis and associations with demographic, disease and lifestyle characteristics: an international cross-sectional study. BMC Neurol. 2016;16(1):210. https://doi.org/10.1186/s12883-016-0735-8. PMID: 27814701; PMCID: PMC5097380.
10. Hadgkiss EJ, Jelinek GA, Weiland TJ, Pereira NG, Marck CH, van der Meer DM. Methodology of an international study of people with multiple sclerosis recruited through Web 2.0 platforms: demographic data, lifestyle and disease characteristics. Neurol Res Int. 2013;2013:580596.
11. Calabro RS, Russo M. Sexual dysfunction and depression in individuals with multiple sclerosis: is there a link? Innov Clin Neurosci. 2015;12(5–6):11–2.
12. Orasanu B, Frasure H, Wyman A, Mahajan ST. Sexual dysfunction in patients with multiple sclerosis. Mult Scler Relat Disord. 2013;2(2):117–23.
13. Lew-Starowicz M, Gianotten WL. Sexual dysfunction in patients with multiple sclerosis. Handb Clin Neurol. 2015;130:357–70.
14. Merghati-Khoei E, Qaderi K, Amini L, Korte JE. Sexual problems among women with multiple sclerosis. J Neurol Sci. 2013;331(1–2):81–5.
15. Celik DB, Poyraz EC, Bingol A, Idiman E, Ozakbas S, Derya K. Sexual dysfunction in multiple sclerosis: gender differences. J Neurol Sci. 2012.
16. Borello-France D, Leng W, O'Leary M, Xavier M, Erickson J, Chancellor MB, et al. Bladder and sexual function among women with multiple sclerosis. Mult Scler. 2004;10:455–61.
17. Gruenwald I, Vardi Y, Gartman I, Juven E, Sprecher E, Yarnitsky D, et al. Sexual dysfunction in women with multiple sclerosis: quantitative sensory testing. Mult Scler. 2007;13:95–105.
18. Sesil Y, Yetimalar Y, Gedizlioglu M, Arpasi E, Tokucoglu F, Kendir AI, et al. Sexual dysfunction and sympathetic skin response recorded from the genital region in women with multiple sclerosis. Mult Scler. 2007;13:742–8.
19. Barret M. Sexuality and multiple sclerosis. 3rd ed. Toronto: MS Society of Canada; 1999.
20. McCabe MP. Relationship functioning and sexuality among people with multiple sclerosis. J Sex Res. 2002;39(4):302–9. https://doi.org/10.1080/00224490209552154.
21. McCabe MP, McKern S, McDonald E, Vowels LM. Changes over time in sexual and relationship functioning of people with multiple sclerosis. J Sex Marital Ther. 2003;29(4):305–21.
22. Zorzon M, Zivadinov R, Monti Bragadin L, Moretti R, De Masi R, Nasuelli D, Cazzato G. Sexual dysfunction in multiple sclerosis: a 2-year follow-up study. J Neurol Sci. 2001;187(1-2):1–5.
23. Schairer L, Foley F, Zemon V, Tyry T, Campagnolo D, Marrie R, et al. The impact of sexual dysfunction on health-related quality of life in people with multiple sclerosis. Mult Scler J. 2013;20(5):610–6.
24. Tudor KI, Eames S, Haslam C, Chataway J, Liechti MD, Panicker JN. Identification of barriers to seeking help for sexual dysfunction in multiple sclerosis. J Neurol. 2018;265(12):2789–802.
25. Foley FW, Zemon V, Campagnolo D, Marrie RA, Cutter G, Tyry T, Beier M, Farrell E, Vollmer T, Schairer L. The Intimacy and Sexuality Questionnaire in Multiple Sclerosis: revalidation and development of a 15-item version with a large US sample. Mult Scler J. 2013;19(9):1197–203.
26. Sanders AS, Foley FW, LaRocca NG, Zemon V. The Multiple Sclerosis Intimacy and Sexuality Questionnaire-19 (MSISQ-19). Sex Disabil. 2000;18:3–24.

27. Carrillo MG, Salas PO, Vergara KR, Cortes Bernal GA, Nava Mesa M, Moreno MK. Tools for the comprehensive evaluation of sexual function in patients with multiple sclerosis. Neurologia. 2020;38(3):197–205.
28. Kaplan TB, Feldman T, Healey B, Behn M, Glanz B, Chitnis T. Sexual problems in MS: sex differences and their impact on quality of life. Mult Scler Relat Disord. 2023;74:104672. https://doi.org/10.1016/j.msard.2023.104672. Epub 2023 Mar 26
29. Gaviria-Carrillo M, Bueno-Florez SJ, Ortiz-Salas PA. Assessment of sexual dysfunction in patients with multiple sclerosis: a perspective from neurologist. BMC Neurol. 2022;22(1):372. https://doi.org/10.1186/s12883-022-02884-y. PMID: 36175888; PMCID: PMC9520880.
30. Rubin R. Communication about sexual problems in male patients with multiple sclerosis. Nurs Stand. 2005;19(24):33–7.
31. Wang G, Marrie RA, Fox RJ, Tyry T, Cofield SS, Cutter GR, et al. Treatment satisfaction and bothersome bladder, bowel, and sexual symptoms in multiple sclerosis. Mult Scler Relat Disord. 2018;20:16–21.
32. Redelman MJ. Sexual difficulties for people with multiple sclerosis in New South Wales, Australia. Int J Rehabil Res. 2009;32(4):337–47.
33. Carotenuto A, De Giglio L, Chiodi A, Petracca M, Rosa L, Bianchi M, Ferrante I, Lauro F, Moccia M, Ianniello A, Pozzilli C, Brescia Morra V, Lanzillo R. Validation of the Italian version of the Multiple Sclerosis Intimacy and Sexuality Questionnaire-19. Neurol Sci. 2021;42(7):2903–10.
34. Printza A, Boziki M, Bakirtzis C, Nikolaidis I, Kalaitzi M, Triaridis S, Grigoriadis N. The modified DYMUS questionnaire is a reliable, valid and easy-to-use tool in the assessment of dysphagia in multiple sclerosis. Eur J Neurol. 2020;27(7):1231–7.
35. Busch AK, Spirig R, Schnepp W. Coping with multiple sclerosis in partnerships: a systematic review of the literature. Nervenarzt. 2014;85(6):727–37. German.
36. Neate SL, Taylor KL, Jelinek GA, De Livera AM, Simpson S Jr, Bevens W, Weiland TJ. On the path together: experiences of partners of people with multiple sclerosis of the impact of lifestyle modification on their relationship. Health Soc Care Community. 2019;27(6):1515–24.
37. Neate SL, Taylor KL, Nag N, Jelinek GA, Simpson-Yap S, Bevens W, Weiland TJ. Views of the future of partners of people with multiple sclerosis who attended a lifestyle modification workshop: a qualitative analysis of perspectives and experiences. Int J Environ Res Public Health. 2020;18(1):85.
38. Rollero C. The experience of men caring for a partner with multiple sclerosis. J Nurs Scholarsh. 2016;48:482–9. https://doi.org/10.1111/jnu.12231.
39. Maguire R, Maguire P. Caregiver burden in multiple sclerosis: recent trends and future directions. Curr Neurol Neurosci Rep. 2020;20(7):18.
40. Merck. Living with multiple sclerosis: the caregiver's perspective. 2018. Available at https://www.merckgroup.com/es-es/informes/Living-with-MS-Carers-Perspective.pdf.
41. Maguire R, Kasilingam E, Kriauzaite N. Caring for children and adolescents with multiple sclerosis: exploring unmet needs and existing supports for pediatric multiple sclerosis caregivers. European Multiple Sclerosis Platform; 2019.
42. Kobelt G, Thompson A, Berg J, Gannedahl M, Eriksson J, Group MS. Platform EMS New insights into the burden and costs of multiple sclerosis in Europe. Mult Scler J. 2017;23(8):1123–36.
43. Hategeka C, Traboulsee A, McMullen K, Lynd LD. Stigma in multiple sclerosis: association with work productivity loss, health-related quality of life, and caregiver burden (P3.332). AAN Enterprises; 2017. https://n.neurology.org/content/88/16_Supplement/P3.332.short.
44. Katsavos S, Artemiadis AK, Zacharis M, Argyrou P, Theotoka I, Chrysovitsanou C, et al. Predicting caregiver status and caregiver burden in multiple sclerosis. A brief report. Neurol Res. 2017;39(1):13–5.
45. Giordano A, Cimino V, Campanella A, Morone G, Fusco A, Farinotti M, et al. Low quality of life and psychological well-being contrast with moderate perceived burden in caregivers of people with severe multiple sclerosis. J Neurol Sci. 2016;366:139–45.

46. Perrin PB, Panyavin I, Morlett Paredes A, Aguayo A, Macias MA, Rabago B, et al. An undue burden: gender differences in mental health, health-related quality of life, and social support in Mexican caregivers of multiple sclerosis patients. Behav Neurol. 2015;2015:1–9.
47. Giordano A, Cimino V, Campanella A, Morone G, Fusco A, Farinotti M, et al. Low quality of life and psychological well-being contrasted with moderate perceived burden in caregivers of people with severe multiple sclerosis. J Neurol Sci. 2016;366:139–45.
48. Pooyania S, Lobchuk M, Chernomas W, Marrie RA. Examination of the relationship between the emotional states of family caregivers and their ability to empathize with patients with multiple sclerosis: a pilot study. Int J MS Care. 2016;18(3):122–8. https://doi.org/10.7224/1537-2073.2015-023.
49. Calvo-Perxas L, Vilalta-Franch J, Litwin H, Turro-Garriga O, Mira P, Garre-Olmo J. What seems to matter in public policy and the health of informal caregivers? A cross-sectional study in 12 European countries. PLoS One. 2018;13(3):e0194232. https://doi.org/10.1371/journal.pone.0194232.

HSDD in Patients with Psoriasis

17

Abstract

Psoriasis is a chronic inflammatory dermatosis of uncertain cause classified as a systemic disease based on recent research. It is prevalent in the global adult population at about 2%. This dermatosis often occurs simultaneously with metabolic syndrome, other serious disorders, and is associated with chronic inflammation, immune disorders, genetic factors, and a variety of biologically active substances secreted by adipose tissue (Fernández-Armenteros JM, J Eur Acad Dermatol Venereolo 33:128–135, 2019). Due to these factors, psoriasis patients are at higher risk of obesity, diabetes mellitus, hypertension, dyslipidemia, and atherosclerosis. Furthermore, these diseases increase the likelihood of cardiovascular events (Ryan C and Kirby B, Dermatol Clin 33:41–55, 2015). In addition, previous research indicates that patients suffer from insomnia and experience poor sleep quality (Mann C et al., J Dtsch Dermatol Ges 21:577–584, 2023). The comorbidities mentioned above directly increase the risk of sexual dysfunction (Cirillo L et al., Arch Ital Urol Androl 95:11236, 2023) in both men and women.

Keywords

Psoriasis · Sexual dysfunction · Female Sexual Function Index (FSFI) · International Erectile Function Index (IIEF) · hypoactive sexual desire disorder (HSDD) · Adolescents · partners families · Pain · Alexithymia

17.1 Introduction

Dermatological patients are generally known to be vulnerable to mental distress, including anxiety, depression and mood disorders, largely because skin lesions are easily visible and attract people's attention. The fact that this disease is often long-lasting adds to the emotional stress. Lastly, from a psychological perspective, it is

E. V. Longhi, *Hypoactive Sexual Desire Disorder*,
https://doi.org/10.1007/978-3-032-00659-2_17

clear that psoriasis is associated with hypoactive sexual desire disorder (HSDD) and sexual dysfunctions.

The World Health Organization (WHO) states that *sexual health is not merely the absence of disease or dysfunction but is characterized by physical, emotional, mental, and social well-being related to sexuality*. Regrettably, people rarely discuss this topic [5].

About 45% of female patients with psoriasis report experiencing problems in the sexual sphere. These difficulties are multifactorial, involving psychological, hormonal, and overall health-related issues. Among men, the most common dysfunctions are hypoactive sexual desire and erectile dysfunction, which can have both organic (neurogenic, vascular, hormonal, or pharmacological) and psychological nature.

The physiology of human sexuality relies on the coordinated action of neurotransmitters that either stimulate (dopamine, adrenaline) or inhibit (serotonin, endogenous opioids) the sexual response, as well as hormones such us testosterone, adrenal androgens, estrogens, progesterone. Additionally, the proper functioning of the cardiovascular and nervous systems is essential. Disorder such as hypoactive sexual desire, sexual arousal dysfunction, and orgasmic dysfunction, the relaxation phase, and genital-pelvic pain significantly impair quality of life.

17.2 Psoriasis and Sexuality

The French study by Salle R. et al. [6] recruited patients through the *National Association of Patients Suffering from Psoriatic Dermatitis.*

Forty-one percent (577) of the patients reported having HSDD and sexual dysfunctions (SD) related to psoriasis. Female patients reported significantly more SD than men [387 (44.7%) versus 190%–35%]. *Three hundred and ninety-six (28.1%) patients reported a reduction in the frequency of sexual activity and hypoactive desire*, 207 (14.7%) described a change in sexual practice, and 284 (27.4%) highlighted an absence of sexual activity, without significant differences between women and men.

The main consequence of sexual difficulties for patients were the loss of self-esteem in 627 (44.5%) cases, feelings of guilt in 209 (14.8%) cases, deterioration of couple life in 214 (15.2%) cases, isolation in 260 (18.5%) cases, and frustration.

The main causes of SD turned out to be physical and psychological, in equal proportions. The physical symptoms of psoriasis do not appear to be the only ones responsible for the sexual discomfort reported by patients in their sexual relationships. *This may be due to the discomfort of the patient or the doctor when talking about sexuality because they cannot find the terms to talk about this topic, which is often considered taboo, and due to age or gender differences.* This aspect of the disease should be taken into account by doctors who care for patients with psoriasis, particularly dermatologists.

17.3 The Greater Patient

Like all chronic diseases, psoriasis does not only affect the individual, but **also the partner and the family**.

One study [7] recruited **183** adult patients with psoriasis and their partners. The severity of psoriasis was measured using the *Psoriasis Area and Severity Index*. The patient's quality of life was assessed using the *Dermatology Life Quality Index and the Short Form-12* (SF12). The impact of psoriasis on the partners' quality of life was measured with the *Family Psoriasis* and the SF12. The presence of sexual dysfunction and empathy in partners were evaluated using the Family Psoriasis.

Forty-nine point seven percent of patients had moderate to severe psoriasis.

The severity of the patient's psoriasis and the quality of life of the patient were correlated with the psychological distress of the partner.

The greatest deterioration in quality of life was observed in female patients with moderate to severe psoriasis. The most significant alteration in quality of life observed in female patients with psoriasis, compared to their partners, was not observed in male patients with psoriasis compared to their partners.

There was no relationship between the quality of life of the partner and the age of the patient or with the duration of psoriasis. Most patients, but fewer than half of the partners, reported *sexual dysfunction* ***(SDy) with age as a significantly more important impact factor than the severity of the disease***.

Both the clinical severity of psoriasis and a significant impact on quality of life were associated factors for sexual dysfunction *(SDy) in male partners of women with psoriasis, but not in female partners of men with psoriasis.*

A previous study [8] **has already identified the distress of partners and family members** *of patients suffering from psoriasis.*

The severity of the patients' psoriasis was measured using the Psoriasis Area and Severity Index (PASI), the Dermatology Life Quality Index (DLQI) and the Psoriasis Disability Index (PDI). Subjects had intensive qualitative interviews with a researcher or responded to a postal questionnaire. Both methods identified ways in which their relative's or partner's psoriasis had affected their lives.

Thirty-three subjects were interviewed, and 30 responded via postal questionnaire. Twenty-eight of the 63 subjects were relatives (7 men and 21 women), and 35 were partners (16 men and 19 women). The average age was 51 years.

The 63 patients had an average DLQI of 10, an average PDI of 13.8, and an average PASI of 5.2. **Forty different aspects of impairment of relatives' and partners' quality of life were identified**.

Seventy percent stated that the treatment of their relative or partner meant they had to devote more time to household chores, 57% described psychological pressures, including anxiety, upset, and concern for the patient's future, 55% described social disruption due to embarrassment or the time required for care duties, 44% described limitations in holiday plans, sports, recreational activities, and evening outings, 37% described limitations in daily activities such as shopping, work, and time spent with other family members, 37% felt that their closest relationships had deteriorated, and only 8% described no effect on their quality of life (QoL).

It is of great importance to identify these issues to allow physicians to develop appropriate care strategies, not only for patients with psoriasis but also for their partners and their families.

Qualitative interviews were conducted with 50 relatives and partners of patients attending a university hospital outpatient clinic, with a wide range of dermatological conditions (*n* = 21). Subjects were invited to discuss in detail all the ways in which their lives were affected by living with a patient with a skin disease [9].

The average age of the subjects was 48.1 years, and most were parents (44%) or spouses or partners (44%) of the patients. The age of the patients ranged from 5 months to 84 years. ***Fifty-nine aspects of the relatives' quality of life that had been negatively affected by the patients' skin disease were identified***.

These were categorized into 18 main thematic areas:

Emotional distress (98%), care burden (54%), effect on household chores (42%), social life (48%), holidays (46%), financial aspect (30%), physical well-being (22%), work/study (40%), recreational activities (26%), sleep (20%), food/drinks (12%), restriction of preferred activities (14%), need for support (12%), people's attitudes (10%), dissatisfaction with medical care (14%), effect on sexual life (8%), role of religious faith (8%), and various (16%).

There was no significant difference between male and female participants regarding the main areas of quality of life affected. The median number of main thematic areas reported per family member was five (range 1–10).

17.4 HSDD and Psoriasis in Adolescents

Semi-structured qualitative interviews were also conducted with a sample of *dermatological patients aged between 12 and 19*, who attended the dermatology clinic of a secondary reference center. Participants were invited to speak in detail about all the ways their lives had been affected by their skin disease. The interviews were transcribed verbatim [9].

Thirty-two adolescents participated in the interviews (males = 10, females = 22), with an average age of 15.7 years.

Twenty-eight health-related quality of life themes negatively affected by skin diseases were identified from the interviews, which were grouped into six main health-related quality domains: psychological impact (91% of patients), physical impact (81%), social impact (81%), lifestyle impact (63%), need for support (41%), and education and employment (34%). The number of health-related quality themes affected in each individual varied between 1 and 23.

Moreover, anxiety and depression play a conditioning role in hypoactive desire in adolescents and adults [11].

A comparative study matched **by sex and age** was conducted. Eighty patients with moderate to severe psoriasis and 80 patients in the healthy control group were included. Participants completed the *Massachusetts General Hospital-Sexual Functioning Questionnaire, the Hospital Anxiety and Depression Scale, and the Self-Administered Psoriasis Area and Severity Index*.

Depending on the areas affected by psoriasis, severe sexual dysfunctions and HSDD were highlighted in patients undergoing dermatological therapy. Anxiety and depression were also identified as independent risk factors for sexual dysfunction in patients with moderate to severe psoriasis.

It follows that some components of the sexual response, such as HSDD, depend mainly on psychological factors and are compromised by conditions such as *anxiety and depression*, while others, like erection and orgasm, can be influenced by psychological and physical causes.

Sexual impairment in patients with psoriasis occurs in all components of the sexual response [12]. This suggests that sexual dysfunction in psoriasis must be a consequence of several combined factors.

17.5 Genital Psoriasis and HSDD

Unexpectedly, studies offering an in-depth analysis of the impact of body image changes in dermatological diseases and their effects on sexual function are scarce, particularly considering that changes in body image are practically constant in skin diseases.

The research, in particular by Meeuwis KA et al., [13], involved 1579 patients with genital psoriasis, members of the *Dutch Psoriasis Association*. They completed several self-administered questionnaires: Dermatology Life Quality Index, Sexual Quality of Life Questionnaire for Use in Men, International Index of Erectile Function, Female Sexual Distress Scale, and Female Sexual Function Index.

Patients with genital lesions reported significantly worse quality of life compared to patients without genital lesions.

Discomfort and sexual dysfunction were particularly evident in women, reported respectively by 37.7% and 48.7% of female patients. Sexual discomfort is especially high when the genital area is affected; for this reason, the *attention given to sexual problems by healthcare providers is perceived as insufficient by psoriatic patients*.

It is no coincidence that *genital psoriasis is a neglected manifestation of psoriasis, although it affects numerous patients and has significant effects on sexual quality of life* (SQoL).

In another study by Meeuwis KA et al. [14], patients were treated for at least 1 year at a specialized outpatient research clinic with extensive attention to genital lesions and SQoL. Genital lesions were treated according to a stepwise algorithm.

The first follow-up was scheduled after 6 weeks; subsequent follow-up visits were scheduled every 3 months. At each visit, the severity of psoriasis and SQoL were measured with validated tools. Differences in scores between visits were analyzed by a mixed model for repeated measures. Forty-two patients (Male: Female = 25:17) were included. *All objective and subjective parameters of the severity of genital psoriasis and QoL significantly improved within the first follow-up period of about 6 weeks.*

The study by Ryan C et al. [15] identified the factors associated with the development of *genital psoriasis* and its impact on quality of life and sexual function.

One hundred and thirty-four patients (38%) had genital involvement at the time of the study, while another 224 (63%) had a current and/or previous history of genital involvement. Eighty-seven percent reported itching, 39% pain, 42% dyspareunia, 32% a worsening of *genital psoriasis* after sexual intercourse, and 43% a decrease in the frequency of sexual intercourse.

Among the factors associated with genital psoriasis and HSDD are early age of onset of psoriasis, male sex, involvement of the scalp, inguinal folds, and nail contour.

In fact, patients with genital psoriasis showed greater deterioration in quality of life and sexual health, as determined by the Dermatology Life Quality Index, the Center for Epidemiological Studies-Depression Scale, and the Relationship and Sexuality Scale.

GENIPSO is a prospective French study [16] conducted by private and hospital dermatologists. This study characterized the consecutive inclusion of patients visiting for extragenital psoriasis. The clinical characteristics of psoriasis and genital psoriasis were recorded, and patients were given questionnaires on quality of life and sexual health.

Three hundred and thirty-five of the 776 patients (43.2%) included in the study had genital involvement. All were aware of having genital lesions, but only **135** patients (40%) stated that they had been previously examined. *Genital lesions were associated with male sex, severity of psoriasis, onset age > 20 years, inverse psoriasis, and involvement of the scalp, nails, and external auditory canal, but were not associated with obesity, psoriatic arthritis, or active sexual life.* **Itching was the main symptom**. Genital psoriasis was associated with impairment of quality of life and sexual health according to the *Dermatology Life Quality Index and the Female Sexual Function Index*.

Previously, a national cross-sectional survey [17] focused on the individual and was conducted online in Germany between March and June 2019. A multiple logistic regression model was used to analyze the data. In total, **344** individuals with *psoriasis* participated.

Of these, **198** (57.6%) ***reported having genital psoriasis***, and **261** (75.9%) were at the time of the survey receiving medical treatment.

The duration of psoriasis, overall subjective severity and pain during sex were associated with the avoidance of sexual activities and hypoactive sexual desire disorder (HSDD).

The most common reasons for avoiding sexual activities were "shame", "pain", and "fear of rejection". Sexual discomfort was high in this sample, and a person-centered care approach has yet to be established with an international psychosexual criterion.

17.6 Conclusions

Psoriasis involves evident changes in body image in the form of visible and touchable lesions that can affect any body area. Psoriasis lesions can affect visible regions of the body, and the involvement of such areas has been linked to a significantly compromised quality of life and a significant interference in social relationships. Such lesions are therefore considered severity criteria for deciding the therapeutic approach.

Feelings of stigmatization, shame, low self-esteem, and increased sexual discomfort would specifically arise during sexual activity, and consequently, sexual dysfunction related to ASI involvement is independent of psychological state in terms of anxiety or depression. Therefore, the presence of signs of anxiety and/or depression and ASI involvement could be considered possible risk factors in the link between psoriasis, sexual dysfunction, and HSDD.

The symptom of pain and its consequences should not be overlooked.

Three focus groups and four interviews were conducted in the study by Snyder Amat et al. [17] with 25 patients with psoriasis.

A qualified facilitator used a guide for semi-structured interviews based on a literature review and a theory-based approach. Two researchers independently coded the narratives and reached a consensus on the main themes using *NVivo* software.

Five main themes regarding pain:

1. The perception of pain was illustrated through intense descriptors.
2. Patients identified pain triggers, including self-inflicted triggers.
3. Patients found coping strategies to manage pain, including the suppression of sensory experiences and sexuality.
4. Emotional suffering was primarily linked to the compulsion to continue scratching despite repeated efforts to stop, and the failure of doctors to recognize the weight of the pain, which led to inadequate pain management.
5. Pain led to a clear impact on health-related quality of life in these patients through interference with daily activities, intimate relationships, hypoactive desire, and sleep.

This means that pain can be a significant difficulty for patients with psoriasis. Doctors need to be encouraged to inquire about pain separately from itching and to consider the impacts on their patients' health-related quality of life when determining treatments—excluding quality of life and sexuality.

Moreover, some patients with psoriasis have difficulty expressing their concerns and doctors may need to encourage their patients to share the emotional impacts of psoriasis [18].

Alexithymia, a condition in which patients have difficulty identifying and expressing emotions, can affect *between 20% and 30% of patients affected by psoriasis and has been associated with worse scores of anxiety, depression, and quality* *of life*. Doctors must be able to understand their patients' perspectives despite the brevity of the typical clinical visit.

In fact, the study by Sampogna F et al. [18] determined the prevalence of alexithymia, as defined by a score ≥ 61 on the *20-item Toronto Alexithymia Scale,* in a large sample of patients affected by plaque psoriasis for ≤10 years and eligible for phototherapy or systemic treatment. The secondary objectives were to investigate the relationship between alexithymia and clinical and psychological aspects of psoriasis.

The data were collected as part of an observational, multicenter, and international study—the Epidemiological Study on Patients with Recently Diagnosed Psoriasis (**PIDEPSO**)—which aimed to investigate the prevalence of alexithymia and other psychosocial comorbidities in patients with psoriasis with disease duration ≤10 years.

The prevalence of alexithymia in a cohort of 670 patients was 24.8%.

Patients with alexithymia had a greater burden of psoriasis, including a significant deterioration in quality of life, hypoactive sexual desire disorder (HSDD), higher levels of anxiety and depression, a higher risk of alcohol dependence, and deterioration of work productivity compared to patients without alexithymia.

It is important to identify alexithymic patients with *psoriasis* in clinical practice, as they are subjects with a higher disease burden and a lower ability to express their feelings.

Once all these components have been identified, it is essential to set up individualized care and psychosexual counseling projects for the patient, the partner, and the family.

References

1. Fernández-Armenteros JM, Gómez-Arbonés X, Buti-Soler M, Betriu-Bars A, Sanmartin-Novell V, Ortega-Bravo M, et al. Psoriasis, metabolic syndrome, and cardiovascular risk factors. A population-based study. J Eur Acad Dermatol Venereol. 2019;33:128–35.
2. Ryan C, Kirby B. Psoriasis is a systemic disease with multiple cardiovascular and metabolic comorbidities. Dermatol Clin. 2015;33:41–55.
3. Mann C, Gorai S, Staubach-Renz P, Goldust M. Sleep disorders in dermatology: a comprehensive review. J Dtsch Dermatol Ges. 2023;21:577–84.
4. Cirillo L, Fusco GM, Di Bello F, Morgera V, Cacace G, Di Mauro E, et al. Sexual dysfunction: is it time for a multidisciplinary approach? Arch Ital Urol Androl. 2023;95:11236.
5. Sexual and Reproductive Health and Research (SRH). Definition of sexual health: report of a technical consultation on sexual health. Geneva: WHO; 2002. Available at: https://www.who.int/teams/sexual-and-reproductive-health-andresearch/key-areas-of-work/sexual-health/defining-sexual-health
6. Salle R, Halioua B, Le Fur G, Aubert R, Shourick J, Taieb C. Psoriasis and sexuality: patients express their feelings. Skin Health Dis. 2022;3(3):e199.
7. Halioua B, Maccari F, Fougerousse AC, Parier J, Reguiai Z, Taieb C, Esteve E. Impact of patient psoriasis on partner quality of life, sexuality and empathy feelings: a study in 183 couples. J Eur Acad Dermatol Venereol. 2020;34(9):2044–50.
8. Eghlileb AM, Davies EE, Finlay AY. Psoriasis has a major secondary impact on the lives of family members and partners. Br J Dermatol. 2007;156(6):1245–50.

9. Basra MK, Finlay AY. The family impact of skin diseases: the greater patient concept. Br J Dermatol. 2007;156(5):929–37.
10. Golics CJ, Basra MK, Finlay AY, Salek MS. Adolescents with skin disease have specific quality of life issues. Dermatology. 2009;218(4):357–66.
11. Molina-Leyva A, Almodovar-Real A, Carrascosa JC, Molina-Leyva I, Naranjo-Sintes R, Jimenez-Moleon JJ. Distribution pattern of psoriasis, anxiety and depression as possible causes of sexual dysfunction in patients with moderate to severe psoriasis. An Bras Dermatol. 2015;90(3):338–45.
12. McMahon CG, Jannini E, Waldinger M, Rowland D. Standard operating procedures for orgasm and ejaculation disorders. J Sex Med. 2013;10:204–29.
13. Meeuwis KA, de Hullu JA, van de Nieuwenhof HP, Evers AW, Massuger LF, van de Kerkhof PC, et al. Quality of life and sexual health in patients with genital psoriasis. Br J Dermatol. 2011;164:1247–55.
14. Meeuwis KA, de Hullu JA, IntHout J, Hendriks IM, Sparreboom EE, Massuger LF, van de Kerkhof PC, van Rossum MM. Genital psoriasis awareness program: physical and psychological care for patients with genital psoriasis. Acta Derm Venereol. 2015;95(2):211–6.
15. Ryan C, Sadlier M, De Vol E, Patel M, Lloyd AA, Day A, Lally A, Kirby B, Menter A. Genital psoriasis is associated with significant impairment in quality of life and sexual functioning. J Am Acad Dermatol. 2015;72(6):978–83.
16. Larsabal M, Ly S, Sbidian E, Moyal-Barracco M, Dauendorffer JN, Dupin N, Richard MA, Chosidow O, Beylot-Barry M. GENIPSO: a French prospective study assessing instantaneous prevalence, clinical features and impact on quality of life of genital psoriasis among patients consulting for psoriasis. Br J Dermatol. 2019;180(3):647–56.
17. Schielein MC, Tizek L, Schuster B, Ziehfreund S, Biedermann T, Zink A. Genital psoriasis and associated factors of sexual avoidance – a people-centered cross-sectional study in Germany. Acta Derm Venereol. 2020;100(10):adv00151.
18. Sampogna F, Puig L, Spuls P, et al. Prevalence of alexithymia in patients with psoriasis and its association with disease burden: a multicenter observational study. Br J Dermatol. 2017;176(5):1195–203.

Polycystic Ovary Syndrome and HSDD

18

Abstract

Polycystic ovary syndrome (PCOS) is a prevalent endocrine and metabolic disorder that occurs in approximately 6–20% of women of reproductive age. Most of the symptoms of PCOS manifest early during puberty. The most accepted diagnostic criterion is the Rotterdam criterion, which includes two of the last three characteristics: hyperandrogenism, oligo- or an-ovulation, and polycystic ovaries. The persistent hormonal imbalance leads to the formation of multiple small antral follicles and an irregular menstrual cycle, causing infertility and HSDD. Additionally, cardiovascular diseases, abdominal obesity, psychological disorders, infertility, and cancer are related to PCOS. Hyperandrogenism then causes insulin resistance and hyperglycemia, leading to the formation of reactive oxygen species (ROS), oxidative stress, and abdominal adiposity. Consequently, there is also an increase in inflammation, ROS production, insulin resistance, and hyperandrogenemia (Siddiqui et al., J Assist Reprod Genet. 39:2439–2473, 2022).

Although the etiology of this disorder is not clear, environmental and genetic factors are mainly involved. Physical inactivity, as well as poor eating habits, play a key role in the progression of PCOS.

The initiation of antiandrogen treatment at an early age (≤25 years) could be helpful in spontaneous conception in women with PCOS.

Keywords

Sexual health · Reproductive health · Advanced glycation end products (AGE) · Antiandrogen treatment · Bone morphogenetic proteins (BMP) · Low-grade chronic inflammation · growth differentiation factor 8 (GDF8) · Genetics · Hyperandrogenism · Insulin resistance · Kisspeptin · Metformin · Oxidative stress · Polycystic ovary syndrome · Serpine1

E. V. Longhi, *Hypoactive Sexual Desire Disorder*,
https://doi.org/10.1007/978-3-032-00659-2_18

18.1 Introduction

One of the key aspects of women's lives is sexual and reproductive health (SRH). According to Reproductive Health (World Health Organization), reproductive health is defined as the state of physical, mental, and social well-being of the reproductive system.

Worldwide, among women of reproductive age, polycystic ovary syndrome (PCOS) is the most common endocrine disorder, significantly affecting reproductive health. Its prevalence in different regions varies between 2.2% and 26%. The syndrome is often associated with insulin resistance, obesity, and hypoactive sexual desire disorder (HSDD) [2]. PCOS can affect the reproductive, metabolic, and endocrine systems, leading to menstrual disorders, endometrial hyperplasia, abnormal uterine bleeding, oligo-ovulation, infertility, and a significant reduction in quality of life. Identifying SRH aspects is necessary to create a comprehensive and effective health plan [3]. Although some studies have evaluated some aspects of SRH, such as infertility, sexual disorders, pregnancy complications, and quality of life for women with PCOS [8–10], no comprehensive study has evaluated all SRH aspects in women with PCOS.

Lifestyle therapy tends to be the first step in managing PCOS, especially when there is excess body weight. Pharmacotherapy is often used to manage the most predominant manifestations in each age group, such as irregular menstruation and hirsutism in adolescence, fertility problems in adulthood, and metabolic problems, HSDD, and cancer risk in older adults.

18.2 Sexual Dysfunctions

Sexual dysfunction, HSDD, occurs at any stage of sexual performance or at any period of the sexual response cycle, but polycystic ovary syndrome (*Polycystic Ovary Syndrome*) affects self-image with repercussions on sexuality.

The study by Firmino Murgel AC et al. [4], conducted a systematic review following the Preferred Reporting Items for Systematic Reviews and Meta-Analysis. The primary databases—*MEDLINE, EMBASE, Cochrane*, and *Lilacs*—were consulted using specific terms. There was no constraint for the year of publication. The meta-analysis was conducted with the RevMan version 5.3 program.

The systematic review included 19 studies. The analysis indicated that 11 specific tools and 6 general ones were used to measure sexual function in women with PCOS. Of these, the *Female Sexual Function Index* was used most frequently. All studies evaluated different aspects of sexual performance in women with PCOS, and no difference was found between women with PCOS and subjects in the control group, except for HSDD, which is predominant in patients with PCOS.

It was also found that these patients—if obese—report more sexual dysfunctions and an almost permanent HSDD.

The study by Ferraresi SR et al. [5] used a cross-sectional study design to evaluate 83 *women, including 19 non-obese women without PCOS, 24 non-obese women* *with PCOS, 16 obese women without PCOS, and 24 obese women with PCOS. The FSFI questionnaire was used to collect data from all women, and free testosterone levels were determined and used to calculate free androgen index (FAI) values. Higher androgen concentrations were evident in the PCOS groups compared to the control groups. This was also true for FAI, except for the control group of obese patients and non-obese women with PCOS, in which the levels were similar. The evaluation of total FSFI scores revealed that obese women without PCOS had below-normal sexual function scores, while both obese and non-obese women with PCOS had borderline scores compared to controls, which had normal FSFI results.*

To conclude, obese women in the sample were at higher risk of sexual dysfunction and lower FSFI scores, and women with PCOS had borderline FSFI values, regardless of their obesity status. It also appears that the somatic characteristics of patients with PCOS, both obese and non-obese, predict ongoing sexual functioning and HSDD.

The study by Zueff LN et al. [6] *sought to predict sexual functioning among 87 sexually active obese women with and without polycystic ovary syndrome (PCOS), aged between 18 and 40 years, and divided into two groups: obese women (44) or obese women with polycystic ovary syndrome (PCOS) (43). The groups were compared using the Sexual Quotient-Female version and the Hospital Anxiety and Depression scales, and through serum tests. No significant difference was observed between the groups in terms of weight, waist-hip ratio, body mass index, blood glucose, cholesterol, triglycerides, total testosterone, sex hormone-binding globulin, total sexual quotient-female version score, and total score ≤60 (risk of sexual dysfunction), as well as hospital anxiety and depression.*

A significant difference was observed in terms of age, parity, and free androgen index. Each unit increase in the waist-hip ratio conferred a higher likelihood of a score ≤60. A height less than 161 cm and the presence of depression were considered risk factors with a score ≤60.

Women with a score ≤60 had significantly smaller hip measurements and waist-hip ratios. The presence of polycystic ovary syndrome was not a risk factor for a reduction in sexual functionality but for HSDD.

It is certain that the undesired body image of patients with polycystic ovary syndrome appears to be a major conditioning factor on sexuality and HSDD.

The study by Kogure GS et al. [7] *studied 94 women of reproductive age who were distinguished based on body mass index (BMI) and sexual function. Data were collected using the Female Sexual Function Index (FSFI), the Body Shape Questionnaire (BSQ), the Figure Rating Scale (FRS), the Hospital Anxiety and Depression Scale (HADS-A and HADS-D), and anthropometric indices. Women with PCOS had self-image perceptual distortions independent of sexual function and BMI.*

There were negative correlations between HADS-A and HADS-D scores and the total FSFI score, while HADS-D scores had positive correlations with weight, anthropometric indices, and the total BSQ score. The degree of dissatisfaction was a predictor of the total FSFI score. Depression and anxiety, HSDD, and the total FSFI score were predicted by HADS-D. Desired and ideal gender BMI were risk factors for sexual dysfunction, and overweight and obesity were risk factors for the degree of dissatisfaction. It can therefore be stated that perception and cognitive-affective dimensions seem to play an important role in body image dysfunction in women with PCOS, in HSDD, and have an impact on sexual dysfunction and depression associated with the syndrome.

These conclusions seem similar in many studies. This is confirmed by the study by Çetinkaya Altuntaş S et al. [8], *which involved 167 women of reproductive age with PCOS and 73 healthy patients from the control group. All participants were administered standardized scales for the evaluation of depression (the Beck Depression Inventory [BDI]), depression and anxiety (the Hospital Anxiety and Depression Scale [HADS] and the General Health Questionnaire [GHQ]) and a body image scale (the Body Cathexis Scale [BCS]). Hirsutism scores, serum levels of androgens and metabolic parameters were recorded.*

Higher BDI, HADS depression, and GHQ scores, as well as a more negative body image in terms of BCS scores, were observed in women with PCOS compared to healthy controls.

BDI scores were significantly higher in phenotypes A, B, and D compared to healthy controls. No significant difference was observed in BDI and HADS depression scores among the phenotypes. Significant differences were only observed between phenotype A and the control group in terms of HADS depression and GHQ scores.

BCS scores were significantly higher in phenotypes A, B, and C compared to healthy controls. No significant difference was determined in the Female Sexual Function Index (FSFI) scores between the PCOS phenotypes and healthy controls.

When all participants were divided into three groups based on body mass index (BMI), a statistically significant difference was only observed between the lean groups of phenotype a (BMI: 18.5–24.9 kg/m^2) and the control group in terms of BDI, HADS depression, and BCS scores.

BDI, HADS depression, and GHQ scores were all higher in patients with PCOS, HSDD, compared to the healthy control group. These characteristics were more pronounced in phenotypes A and B, including hyperandrogenism and oligo-anovulation.

18.3 Psyche and Sexuality

Clinical signs such as *hirsutism, acne, alopecia, HSDD, seborrhea* along with obesity and infertility, can cause a significant amount of emotional distress [9]. These physical, physiological, and psychological changes can cause mood disorders, including a significant reduction in quality of life, lower self-esteem, and marital and social maladjustments [10].

In addition to high levels of *anxiety and tension leading to depression, eating disorders, and sexual dysfunction* [11].

After approval from the *Tarbiat Modares University Medical Ethics Committee* (IR.MODARES.REC.1397.153), a study was conducted on **242** sexually active participants aged between 18 and 40 years (85% of women with PCOS were infertile and 60% were obese) [12].

The study group included women with PCOS referred to an infertility clinic at Arash Hospital in Tehran province, Iran, from May 2018 to February 2019. The control group also included patients referred to Arash Hospital, in line with healthy and fertile married women, who were not pregnant, not breastfeeding, without PCOS (or other serious gynecological conditions, such as endometriosis or chronic diseases) and with a regular menstrual cycle.

The inclusion criteria were: age between 18 and 40 years, married, not pregnant, of Iranian descent, and personal consent to participate in the study. For the PCOS group, completion of primary school as a minimum level of education and no medication with hormones known to affect serum androgen levels, including anti-androgen drugs and oral contraceptive pills during the 3 months prior to the study, were required. Due to the effects of the medication on the results, patients taking metformin for PCOS (not for high blood glucose level) were excluded.

Those participants who were not eligible for the study—such as those with thyroid dysfunction, abnormal prolactin levels, congenital adrenal hyperplasia (CAH), Cushing's syndrome (CS), androgen-secreting tumors, or diagnosed cardiovascular diseases (CVD)—as well as those taking oral contraceptives and anti-androgen drugs, were excluded from this study.

According to the results obtained, in the FSFI questionnaire, significant differences were observed in arousal, lubrication, HSDD, pain, and total FSFI scores between the different PCOS phenotypes and the control group.

It was also found that the sexual symptom scores in phenotype B were significantly lower compared to the other phenotypes and the control group, which corresponded to the study of Bazarganipoor et al. [13], who reported higher sexual dysfunctions in the group with menstrual irregularities and HSDD. *These results can be explained by the hormonal difference*. It seems that a high level of luteinizing hormone (LH) can cause increased synthesis of androgens, and the increase in circulating androgen levels leads to various virilizing changes, including clitoromegaly, hirsutism, acne, alopecia, HSDD.

In a national survey in Germany, using the SF-12 scale, Benson et al. [14] found that *women with PCOS were at a higher risk of common psychiatric disorders, such as anxiety, depression, or both, which correlated with a lower health-related quality of life (HRQL).*

Another study by Bazarganipoor et al. [13], using *the SF-36 scale, showed that the psychological dimension was more affected than the physical dimension was more affected than the physical domain, and psychological deterioration was higher in patients with HA and menstrual irregularities compared to the other two phenotypes.*

Moran et al., who compared different PCOS phenotypes based on the criteria of the National Institute of Health (NIH) (HA and OD), reported poorer health-related quality of life in women with NIH PCOS compared to women with non-NIH PCOS. Moreover, they found that anxiety and depression levels were similar in women with NIH and non-NIH PCOS.

The relationship between sexual function, anxiety, depression, and infertility remains controversial.

In a study conducted by Diamond et al. [15], it was confirmed that sexual function in women with PCOS did not differ from those without PCOS, and similarly, there was no significant difference in sexual function between women with infertility. Kukur Suna K et al. [16] reported that sexual dysfunction was identical between infertile women and healthy women, but depression scores were higher in infertile women compared to the control group, which is consistent with the results of our study.

Furthermore, Monga et al. [17] did not report any significant difference in sexual function between the infertile group and the fertile group, but the quality of life in the infertile group was lower than that of the fertile group.

These results are contrary to the findings of Deniz et al., [18], who reported that ***women affected by Polycystic Ovary Syndrome and infertility had more problems in all subscales of sexual function and desire, except for arousal, indicating that infertility represents a significant risk of sexual dysfunction in women affected by PCOS*** [19].

The most recent results shared in the scientific literature have revealed a significant observed relationship between age and sexual function, and with an increase of 1 year of age, the possibility of developing sexual dysfunction increased by 8.5%.

Bancroft et al. [20] found that this discomfort for the relationship and one's own sexuality is common in women aged between 20 and 65 years.

There is a general agreement in the literature that, with increasing age, there is a decrease in sexual desire and interest.

The study by Laumann showed that anxiety about sexual function decreased with increasing age [21], and similar results were published by Richter's: while anxiety during sex remained constant with age, concern about attractiveness decreased [22].

18.4 Sexuality in Stable Heterosexual Couples

The study by Warchala A et al. [23] recruited 160 patients divided into two groups: 91 women with *Polycystic Ovary Syndrome* and their partners, and 69 women without *Polycystic Ovary Syndrome* and their partners as a control group.

The *Changes in Sexual Functioning Questionnaire 14* (CSFQ-14) was used to assess sexual dysfunction. The CSFQ-14 measures overall sexual functioning (sum of 1–14 items), with five subdomains that evaluate pleasure (Item 1), desire/frequency (Items 2 and 3), desire/interest (Items 4–6), arousal (Items 7–9) and orgasm (Items 11–13).

Seven questions were asked using the *Visual Analogue Scale* (VAS) [24]:

- How important is a satisfying sexual life to you?
- How many sexual thoughts and fantasies have you had in the past?
- Do you find yourself sexually attractive?

- How does excessive body hair affect your sexuality?
- Does your appearance make it difficult to establish social contacts?
- In the last 4 weeks, how often have you experienced pain during intercourse?
- How satisfied have you been with your sexual life in the last 4 weeks?

Most participants reported having higher or secondary education and a stable job, while 12 partners were unemployed, and four were receiving a pension.

In terms of pleasure, desire (interest), orgasm, and total score, the analysis showed a statistically significant difference between women and their partners

The pattern of differences between women and men was similar in both the *Polycystic Ovary Syndrome* group and the control group, suggesting higher levels of pleasure, desire (interest), orgasm, and overall sexual functioning reported by men, regardless of the presence or absence of a *Polycystic Ovary Syndrome* diagnosis in their partners.

Pastoor et al. [24] demonstrated that women with *Polycystic Ovary Syndrome* experienced *Female Sexual Dysfunction* (FSD) in terms of *Hypoactive Sexual Desire Disorder* (HSDD), arousal, lubrication, sexual satisfaction, orgasm, and overall scores, when compared to control groups.

However, Zhao et al. demonstrated that there are no statistically significant differences in FSD between women with Polycystic Ovary Syndrome and women without this diagnosis [25]. Moreover, Loh et al. [26] conducted the most extensive meta-analysis and found that women with Polycystic Ovary Syndrome have a 30% higher risk of developing FSD compared to women without it. *They confirmed that the total scores of the Female Sexual Function Index (FSFI) did not differ significantly between the study group and the control group, while women with Polycystic Ovary Syndrome scored significantly lower in the pain and satisfaction subscales, compared to control groups. In their opinion, this indicated limitations in the use of this scale to assess sexual desire and the overlap between desire and arousal* [27].

Regardless of the limitations of the FSFI, it is important to remember that both men and women may have difficulty distinguishing between desire and arousal because sexual stimuli trigger both desire and arousal simultaneously [28].

Evaluation of individual sexual domains leads to the conclusion that women with Polycystic Ovary Syndrome derive significantly less satisfaction from their sexual life compared to women without this syndrome [29].

This may be due to specific symptoms such as hyperandrogenism, hirsutism, and oligo- or anovulation, characteristic of phenotypes A and B [30].

These symptoms have negative impacted physical appearance, resulting in a decreased perception of "female identity" and a feeling of "poor attractiveness" [31], as well as a deterioration of "self-image" and reduced "self-esteem" [32].

Furthermore, as the impact of excessive hair on sexuality (VAS4) and the social problems related to appearance (VAS5) increase, the level of pleasure decreases. Additionally, higher scores on the Ferriman-Gallwey scale worsen the perceived impact of excessive hair on sexuality (VAS4). Ercan et al. reported a significant negative correlation between total FSFI scores and total and free testosterone levels [33]. Veras et al. showed a negative correlation between sexual functions and levels of total testosterone and dehydroepiandrosterone sulfate [9].

18.5 Conclusions

Multidisciplinary care models should offer integrated care with personalized therapies, education, and lifestyle support, as well as treatment. Healthcare for this patient group should include not only gynecologists, endocrinologists, general practitioners, dietitians, and exercise physiologists, but also guarantee open access to psychologists and sexologists. Including the partner's continual involvement can facilitate the development of a shared sexual contract according to the needs and wants of both individuals. This can enhance patient-caregiver interaction and support [34, 35].

Finally, the study by Thannickal A et al. [36] collected comprehensive research, including *MEDLINE*, *Embase*, *Cochrane Central Register of Controlled Trials*, *Cochrane Database of Systematic Reviews*, and *Scopus* up to August 1, 2018, reporting the prevalence of *eating disorders, sleep disorders, or sexual function disorders in patients with Polycystic Ovary Syndrome* (PCOS).

Included were **36** studies reporting **349,529 patients**. Compared to women without Polycystic Ovary Syndrome, women with it were more likely to have bulimia nervosa, binge eating or any eating disorder but not anorexia nervosa. Women with Polycystic Ovary Syndrome were more likely to have sleep disorders such as hypersomnia and obstructive sleep apnea. They also had lower sexual satisfaction and desire, measured on a visual analog scale, but showed no difference in the total Female Sexual Function Index.

In practice, Hypoactive Sexual Desire Disorder (HSDD) can be addressed as an index of multidisciplinary pathology of heterogeneous nature: biological, intrapsychic, relational, and social factors, all significantly altering the quality of life of patients with Polycystic Ovary Syndrome.

References

1. Siddiqui S, Mateen S, Ahmad R, Moin S. A brief insight into the etiology, genetics, and immunology of polycystic ovarian syndrome (PCOS). J Assist Reprod Genet. 2022;39(11):2439–73.
2. Bellver J, Rodríguez-Tabernero L, Robles A, Muñoz E, Martínez F, Landeras J, et al. Polycystic ovary syndrome throughout a woman's life. J Assist Reprod Genet. 2018;35:25–39.
3. Singh S, Darroch JE, Ashford LS. Adding it up: the costs and benefits of investing in sexual and reproductive health 2014. New York: Guttmacher Institute; 2016.
4. Firmino Murgel AC, Santos Simões R, Maciel GAR, Soares JM Jr, Baracat EC. Sexual dysfunction in women with polycystic ovary syndrome: systematic review and meta-analysis. J Sex Med. 2019;16(4):542–50.
5. Ferraresi SR, Lara LA, Reis RM, Rosa e Silva AC. Changes in sexual function among women with polycystic ovary syndrome: a pilot study. J Sex Med. 2013;10(2):467–73.

6. Zueff LN, Lara LA, Vieira CS, Martins Wde P, Ferriani RA. Body composition characteristics predict sexual functioning in obese women with or without PCOS. J Sex Marital Ther. 2015;41(3):227–37.
7. Kogure GS, Ribeiro VB, Lopes IP, Furtado CLM, Kodato S, Silva de Sá MF, Ferriani RA, Lara LADS, Maria Dos Reis R. Body image and its relationships with sexual functioning, anxiety, and depression in women with polycystic ovary syndrome. J Affect Disord. 2019;253:385–93.
8. Çetinkaya Altuntaş S, Çelik Ö, Özer Ü, Çolak S. Depression, anxiety, body image scores, and sexual dysfunction in patients with polycystic ovary syndrome according to phenotypes. Gynecol Endocrinol. 2022;38(10):849–55.
9. Veras AB, Bruno RV, de Avila MA, Nardi AE. Sexual dysfunction in patients with polycystic ovary syndrome: clinical and hormonal correlations. Compr Psychiatry. 2011;52:486–9.
10. Jones GL, Hall JM, Ledger WL. Measuring health-related quality of life in women with polycystic ovary syndrome: a systematic review. Hum Reprod Update. 2008;14:15–25.
11. Himelein MJ, Thatcher SS. Polycystic ovary syndrome and mental health: a review. Obstet Gynecol Surv. 2006;61:723–32.
12. Bahadori F, Jahanian Sadatmahalleh S, Montazeri A, Nasiri M. Sexuality and psychological well-being in different polycystic ovary syndrome phenotypes compared with healthy controls: a cross-sectional study. BMC Womens Health. 2022;22(1):390.
13. Bazarganipour F, Ziaei S, Montazeri A, Foroozanfard F. Predictive factors of health-related quality of life in patients with polycystic ovary syndrome: a structural equation modeling approach. Fertil Steril. 2013;100(5):1389–96.
14. Benson S, Hahn S, Tan S, Mann K, Janssen O. Prevalence and implication of anxiety in polycystic ovary syndrome: results of an Internet-based survey in Germany. Hum Reprod Update. 2009;24:1446–51.
15. Diamond M, Righard S, Michael P, Christos CL. Sexual function in infertile women with polycystic ovary syndrome and unexplained infertility. Am J Obstet Gynecol. 2017;17:378–85.
16. Kukur Suna K, Llay G, Aysenur A, Kerem HG. Effect of infertility etiology and depression on female sexual function. J Sex Marital Ther. 2016;42:27–35.
17. Monga M, Alexandrescu B, Katz S, Stein M. Impact of infertility on quality of life, marital adjustment, and sexual function. Urology. 2004;63(1):126–30.
18. Deniz A, Kehribar L. Evaluation of sexual function in infertile women with polycystic ovary syndrome. Niger J Clin Pract. 2020;23:1548–54.
19. Longhi EV. Framing sexual dysfunctions and diseases during fertility treatment. Springer; 2025.
20. Bancroft J, Loftus J, Long JS. Distress about sex: a survey national on women in heterosexual relationships. Arch Sex Behav. 2003;32:193–208.
21. Laumann EPA, Rosen R. Sexual dysfunction in the United States. JAMA. 1999;281:537–44.
22. Richters J, Grulich A, Rissel C, Visser RO, Smith AMA, Rissel CE. Sex in Australia: autoerotic, esoteric and other sexual practices performed by a representative sample of adults. Aust NZJ Public Health. 2003;27:180–90.
23. Warchala A, Madej P, Kochanowicz M, Krzystanek M. Sexual function in women with polycystic ovary syndrome living in stable heterosexual relationships: a cross-sectional study. J Clin Med. 2024;13(8):2227.
24. Pastoor H, Timman R, de Klerk C, Bramer WM, Laan ET, Laven JS. Sexual function in women with polycystic ovary syndrome: a systematic review and meta-analysis. Reprod Biomed Online. 2018;37:750–60.
25. Zhao S, Wang J, Xie Q, Luo L, Zhu Z, Liu Y, Luo J, Zhao Z. Is polycystic ovary syndrome associated with the risk of female sexual dysfunction? A systematic review and meta-analysis. Reprod Biomed Online. 2019;38:979–89.
26. Loh HH, Yee A, Loh HS, Kanagasundram S, Francis B, Lim LL. Sexual dysfunction in polycystic ovary syndrome: a systematic review and meta-analysis. Hormones. 2020;19:413–23.
27. Forbes MK, Baillie AJ, Schniering CA. Critical defects in the female sexual function index and the international index of erectile function. J Sex Res. 2014;51:485–91.
28. Brotto LA, Heiman JR, Tolman DL. Narratives of desire in middle-aged women with and without arousal difficulties. J Sex Res. 2009;46:387–98.

29. Stapinska-Syniec A, Grabowska K, Szpotanska-Sikorska M, Pietrzak B. Depression, sexual satisfaction and other psychological issues in women with polycystic ovary syndrome. Gynecol Endocrinol. 2018;34:597–600.
30. Tian X, Ruan X, Du J, Cheng J, Ju R, Mueck AO. Sexual function in Chinese women with different clinical phenotypes of polycystic ovary syndrome. Gynecol Endocrinol. 2023;39:2221736.
31. Morotti E, Persico N, Battaglia B, Fabbri R, Meriggiola MC, Venturoli S, Battaglia C. Body imaging and sexual behavior in slim women with polycystic ovary syndrome. J Sex Med. 2013;10:2752–60.
32. Sills ES, Perloe M, Tucker MJ, Kaplan CR, Genton MG, Schattman GL. Diagnostic and therapeutic characteristics of polycystic ovary syndrome: descriptive measurements of patient perception and awareness from 657 self-reported cases. BMC Womens Health. 2001;1:3.
33. Ercan CM, Coksuer H, Aydogan U, Alanbay I, Keskin U, Karasahin KE, Baser I. Evaluation of sexual dysfunction and hormonal correlations in patients with polycystic ovary syndrome. Int J Impot Res. 2013;25:127–32.
34. Joham AE, Norman RJ, Stener-Victorin E, Legro RS, Franks S, Moran LJ, Boyle J, Teede HJ. Polycystic ovary syndrome. Lancet Diabetes Endocrinol. 2022;10:668–80. https://doi.org/10.1016/S2213-8587(22)00163-2. Erratum in Lancet Diabetes Endocrinol. 2022, 10, e11.
35. Longhi EV. Managing psychosexual consequences in chronic diseases. Springer; 2024.
36. Thannickal A, Brutocao C, Alsawas M, Morrow A, Zaiem F, Murad MH, Javed Chattha A. Eating, sleeping and sexual function disorders in women with polycystic ovary syndrome (PCOS): a systematic review and meta-analysis. Clin Endocrinol. 2020;92(4):338–49.

Part V

Broader Perspectives and Emerging Topics

HSDD and COVID-19: An Epidemic That Has Undermined the Sense of Desire and Sexual Pleasure

19

Abstract

During the COVID-19 coronavirus epidemic, the psychological burden on each individual affected sexual desire and function. The negative effects of COVID-19 were felt even by those who did not contract the disease. In particular, measures to prevent the disease drastically reduced communication and interpersonal contact. Additionally, people experienced a significant decline in the desire for intimacy due to fear of infection. The lack of comprehensive and updated information on the sexual status of married and single individuals has prompted considerable research in this area.

Keywords

Coronavirus · COVID-19 · Sexual behavior · Sexual dysfunctions · Sexual health · Internet · Healthcare providers

19.1 Introduction

Scientific literature has investigated the consequences of the COVID-19 pandemic during its course in various countries.

Among these, a cross-sectional study was conducted online by Yekefallah L et al. [1] on 400 married individuals residing in Qazvin, Iran, from October 15 to November 12, 2020. The following questionnaires were used for data collection: *Female Sexual Function Index (FSFI), Rosen Male Sexual Function, Larson's Sexual Satisfaction, and Hurlbert Index of Sexual Desire (HISD)*. The questionnaires were sent to participants via online messengers. The results showed that only 19.20% of study participants had sexual intercourse three or more times a week. Most of the female participants (56.90%) had sexual dysfunction, while most of the men (64.30%) reported proper sexual function. Additionally, most participants had moderate sexual desire (46%) and high sexual satisfaction. *The main predictors of*

E. V. Longhi, *Hypoactive Sexual Desire Disorder*,
https://doi.org/10.1007/978-3-032-00659-2_19

sexual dysfunction in men and women during the COVID-19 outbreak were, respectively, "healthcare center workers" and "spouse working in healthcare centers".

The Larson's sexual satisfaction and Hurlbert index of sexual desire (HISD) consists of 25 items to measure sexual desire in both sexes. Each item was rated on a five-point Likert scale (from always = 0 to never = 4). The minimum possible score was 0 and the maximum was 100. *Scores below 50 indicated low sexual desire, 51–75 indicated moderate desire, and 75–100 indicated medium-high desire*.

Among the married participants residing in Qazvin, 112 were men (28%) and 288 were women (72%). The average age of the participants was 36.28.

The sexual function of female participants in this study had a significant direct relationship with poor sexual satisfaction and decreased desire. Similarly, the sexual function of male participants was directly and significantly correlated with sexual satisfaction and higher sexual desire than women.

19.2 Sex, Couples, Individuals, and COVID-19

The results of this study showed that women's sexual function bordered on dysfunction. The findings are consistent with studies by Fuchs et al. [2] on *Polish* women and Culha et al. [3] on Turkish women. The psychological outcomes of the COVID-19 pandemic compromised the sexual function of married women. In contrast, men's sexual function had a desirable status.

Li et al. and Karsiyakali et al. [4] observed a decrease in sexual function during the COVID-19 pandemic, which contradicted the results of previous studies [5]. *The reason for this disparity in results could be due to the pandemic conditions at the time of data collection*. At certain times, the number of people infected with coronavirus increased and the epidemic was at its peak. In these situations, the psychological burden on society was also higher. Cultural differences in societies can influence the expression of sexual issues and research outcomes.

The total sexual satisfaction score in both sexes highlighted moderate sexual satisfaction and low desire during the COVID-19 pandemic. Sexual satisfaction may have decreased compared to the pre-pandemic period, but there is no authentic data source for such a comparison. Karagöz et al. [6] *found a decrease in sexual satisfaction and desire in both male and female subjects during the pandemic. Cocci* et al. [7] *also revealed a decrease in sexual satisfaction during quarantine, with more than half of the respondents expressing complete sexual dissatisfaction. In their study, depression and dissatisfaction with quarantine led to a decrease in sexual satisfaction and desire. There is no doubt that cultural differences also had an impact during the pandemic. Official authorities, such as the New York City government and the Australasian Society for HIV, Viral Hepatitis and Sexual Health Medicine, suggested that partners explore sexual activities without direct physical contact, with masturbation as the safer option. While masturbation could limit the risk of contamination and provide stress relief benefits, solitary sex did not always compensate for partnered sexuality, also causing feelings of guilt, depression, and altered intimate desire. Without drawing general conclusions or ignoring intra- and interpersonal differences in the meaning of pandemic stress for individuals and couples, it has been shown that situations of high stress and prolonged quarantine have induced symptoms of depression, post-traumatic stress, loneliness, confusion, anger, frustration, boredom, worry, and health-related fear* [8]. *The sudden change in daily routine, the limitation of personal and work activities, and spending more time at home increase levels of anxiety and stress. Many people had to change and adapt their roles, for example, shifting from being career-focused to being full-time parents, with little or no opportunity to adjust to this change. Furthermore* [9], *the stress of always being at home and combining different roles meant that some people were able to invest less time in self-care, experienced weight changes, and generally felt less in tune with them, resulting in reduced attraction and sexual desire. These disruptions in identity, along with reduced social contact and limited engagement in valued activities or healthy behaviors unrelated to COVID-19, have caused distress, adding to existing fears about health and the socioeconomic consequences of the COVID-19 crisis. This concern* [10] *for frightening thoughts can distract attention from sexually intimate cues, reducing sexual arousal and perhaps even inducing sexual problems such as genital pain or erectile dysfunction. For single individuals, opportunities to meet a partner were completely lost. For couples living apart, this meant not being able to see their partner for many months. Isolation, travel restrictions, social distancing, and forced cohabitation have had a strong influence on all areas of people's lives, as well as their sexuality. The main objective of Eleuteri S* [11] *was to investigate how the COVID-19 epidemic and its consequences have impacted people's sexuality. In particular, the study focused on:* (1) *the variables associated with the improvement or deterioration of the lives of individuals and couples during the pandemic;* (2) *the use of sex as a coping strategy;* (3) *the impact of the COVID-19 epidemic on LGBT individuals. The results showed that the worsening of sexual life seems to be correlated with conflicts, emotions, and psychological difficulties of couples, being female, being single or away from the partner, being a healthcare worker, and having children. Additionally, a negative effect on sexuality was associated with stress, forced cohabitation, routine, anxiety, and concern about work and the pandemic, feeling distant from the partner, dissatisfaction with the partner, and lack of privacy. On the other hand, improvements in sexuality were associated with a happy life with a partner, being happy and satisfied with a partner, feeling less stressed and more bored, having more free time, fewer leisure opportunities, and having a lighter workload. During the pandemic, there was an increase in the use of sex toys, pornography consumption, masturbation, and attempts at sexual experimentation. Among LGBT individuals, there was an increase in the number of casual sexual partners, potentially due to the perceived lower likelihood of transmission through sex. Additionally, the increase in sexual activity may have represented a coping strategy for quarantine-related distress. The study conducted by Baran and Aykac in 2021* [12] *revealed that Turkish men* had fewer sexual encounters, with lower quality, due to the fear of COVID-19 transmission. Another study [13] reported that most people had unprotected sex and that the prevalence of early-stage syphilis had increased. To date, [14] there is limited data on the impact of coronavirus on individuals' sexual lives, and there are some gaps and conflicting information regarding the effect of COVID-19 on sexual activities, function, and satisfaction.

The effects of COVID-19 on human sexuality have been widely discussed in both mass media [print, radio, and television) and social media (Facebook, YouTube, Instagram, and Twitter; Döring & Walter, [15]]. For example, the *New York Times* published "Coronavirus and Sex: Questions and Answers" [16], *VICE* Magazine reported "How Sex Workers are Dealing with Coronavirus" [17], and a new Facebook group titled "*LGBTI COVID-19 Response*" was founded.

19.3 Surveys During COVID-19

The Kinsey Institute (Indiana University), for example, launched a three-wave longitudinal study on "Sex and Relationships in the Time of COVID-19" (https://kinseyinstitute.org/research/covid-relationships.php) in March 2020. An international network of trans organizations and research institutes initiated a global survey on "Measuring the Impact of the COVID-19 Pandemic on Trans Health and Trans Healthcare" (https://transcarecovid-19.com/). The *Global Network of Sex Work Projects* (NSWP) launched an international survey on the perceptions of sex workers and sex work organizations regarding the effects of COVID-19 in April 2020 (https://www.nswp.org/news/nswp-launch-covid-19-impact-survey). In Germany, for instance, in collaboration with the *German Institute for Sexual Pedagogy*, sexual educators were surveyed about their working conditions during the pandemic (https://www.tu-ilmenau.de/en/media-psychology-and-media-design/research/corona-survey/).

Literature reviews show that mental health significantly deteriorated after the 2008 economic crisis [18] and during quarantine measures related to previous pandemics [19]. An increase in anger, anxiety, post-traumatic stress symptoms, depression, or even suicidal tendencies usually had a negative impact on relationships and sexual life and could promote sexual dysfunctions and deviations. *Some studies also show that divorce rates increase following natural disasters* [20].

19.4 COVID and Escorts

To leave no data unaddressed: in the city of Surat, in Gujarat, India, targeted interventions (TI) based on female sex workers (FSWs) and community-based organizations (CBOs) have been operational since 1998.

To document the impact of the COVID-19 lockdown (March–May 2020) on FSWs and the preventive measures for STI/RTI/HIV provided through TI/CBO in Surat, a sequential explanatory mixed design was used [21].

A document review of quarterly programmatic data (2018–2020) from four TI and CBO was conducted, and 221 FSWs were interviewed to study the socioeconomic conditions pre- and post-lockdown, engagement in sex work, healthcare services during the COVID-19 lockdown, and coping strategies, followed by five focus group discussions with FSWs and TI/CBO project staff.

The study identified four main themes: reasons for working as FSWs during the COVID-19 lockdown, access to sex work during or as a consequence of the lockdown, exploitation of FSWs during the lockdown, and challenges faced by TIs and CBOs in providing services during pandemic situations.

The presence of a strong TIs/CBOs network facilitated the rapid delivery of essential goods and financial aid to FSWs. However, laboratory and screening services were hindered, justifying the need to introduce self-testing kits. In the context of decreased condom distribution, the continuation of sex work during the lockdown, and the disruption of routine screening facilities for HIV/STI/RTI, screenings for HIV/STI/RTI among FSW were intensified.

19.5 United States, Sex, COVID-19, and the Internet

Studies conducted in the early months of the coronavirus pandemic (COVID-19) and the consequent lockdown and social distancing measures demonstrated a decline in sexual frequency and relationship satisfaction [22]. In the United States, 1051 participants were recruited (in October 2020) to complete an online cross-sectional survey. Participants were asked to retrospectively report the frequency of their sexual behavior, relationship satisfaction, and intimate partner desire during the pandemic and before the pandemic.

There was a minimal but significant decrease in some reported couple sexual activities retrospectively, and men reported an increase in autoeroticism and the use of pornographic material, at the expense of sexual desire.

There was no evidence of a change in relationship satisfaction or intimate partner "violence," but both men and women reported a ***decrease in sexual pleasure and sexual desire***. *The sexual behaviors with the greatest reduction were casual sex and the number of partners mostly without experiencing pleasure*. Symptoms of depression, relationship status, and the perceived importance of social distancing emerged as predictors of these reductions. ***Less than half of the individuals who had engaged in casual sexual encounters before the onset of the pandemic completely ceased this behavior after the pandemic began. Individuals waited an average of 6–7 weeks after the end of the pandemic before resuming casual sex*** [23].

19.6 The Word of the Internet

As of April 2022, there were five billion Internet users worldwide, representing 63% of the global population. Of this total, 4.65 billion were social media users [24]. Additionally, the percentage of adults in the United States using social media increased from 5% in 2005 to 79% in 2019. Young people might spend up to 12 h a day on social platforms [25] such as: Facebook (2.38 billion users) and YouTube, followed in descending order by WhatsApp, WeChat, Instagram, TikTok, Weibo,

Reddit, Twitter, Pinterest, and Snapchat. The popularity of social media platforms varies by age. This is particularly true for Instagram and Snapchat, where the age gradient is very steep [26].

During the lockdown, due to social distancing, meetings, work, education, and social contacts were organized online. The average time spent using the Internet and social media increased significantly. *In 2020, United States users spent 65 minutes per day on social media compared to 54 minutes and 56 minutes in previous years. The data suggest that the development of digital media in recent years has impacted all areas of life* [27].

In 2002, J. Brown et al. [28] conducted a study noting that sexual content in mass media can impact individuals' beliefs and sexual behavior. At the time, people wondered if individuals engaged in sex with multiple partners or without any feelings because they saw this behavior in the media and repeated these patterns. Furthermore, the ***COVID-19 pandemic may have exacerbated this impact.*** The purpose of this study was to investigate the relationship between social media use and female sexuality during the COVID-19 pandemic.

Additionally, social media addiction was measured using the *Bergen Social Media Addiction Scale (BSMAS),* a six-item tool used to assess the risk of social media disorder (SMD) [29].

Problematic social media use (PSMU) was defined as the lack of regulation of social media use by an individual associated with negative outcomes in daily functioning. Previous meta-analyses reported the prevalence of PSMU before the onset of the COVID-19 pandemic.

The study by *Casale S* et al. [30] evaluated 139 samples from independent studies with 133,955 respondents from 32 countries covering seven regions of the world.

The results show that PSMU:

A. Is significantly higher in low-income countries (LIC).
B. Has not increased over the last 7 years in general and after the onset of the COVID-19 pandemic, except for LIC.
C. Did not vary according to age and gender. The higher prevalence of PSMU reported during the COVID-19 pandemic by some individual studies may have been a transient phenomenon to cope with physical distancing in some countries, while in others, there was an overall increase in PSMU.
D. The high levels of PSMU could be explained by socio-cultural differences between countries, but also by the higher prevalence of mental disorders as PSMU could be a symptom of other more primary psychiatric disorders.

19.7 Conclusions

Many factors influenced sexuality and intimate desire during the pandemic. The study by Abedinzadeh M et al. [31] was conducted to **evaluate the effect of the coronavirus on men's sexual activity**. A total of **200** men with COVID-19, confirmed by an oropharyngeal swab, who had recovered from the coronavirus for

3 months, were enrolled. These men completed the *International Index of Erectile Function 5 (IIEF-5)* questionnaire for their current and previous sexual status. Then, based on their IIEF-5 score, ***sexual activity before and after the coronavirus infection was compared***.

The average age of the participants was 31.5 ± 3.2 years. This study showed a significant difference between the mean IIEF-5 scores before and after COVID-19, which were 20.4 and 18.6, respectively (p = 0.000). The condition of 56.1% of patients did not change; however, *the coronavirus had a negative effect on 39.6% of patients*.

Forty-one percent of patients reported an improvement in sexual performance, and 45% did not report erectile dysfunction (ED) before contracting the coronavirus, whereas only 27.7% did not report ED after contracting COVID-19.

The results show that COVID-19 affected the sexual activity of infected men, who also showed a higher prevalence of ED after the COVID-19 infection; however, hormonal assessment should have been observed in the follow-up.

In conclusion, healthcare workers also experienced hypoactive sexual desire and poorer sexual performance.

In this context, the study by *Bulut EC et al.* [32] investigated **159** male healthcare workers working in COVID-19 units and a control group of 200 individuals by having them complete the *Impact of Event Scale-Revised (IES-R) and the Index of Erectile Function 5 (IIEF-5)*.

The group of healthcare workers was divided into subgroups based on occupation (doctor, nurse), age group (18–25, 26–30, >30), marital status, and work unit (suspected patient area, diagnosed patient area). Both stress disorder and erectile dysfunction were observed at higher rates in the healthcare worker group ($p < 0.001$).

The median IIEF-5 scores of nurses, married subjects, and those working in the diagnosed patient area were higher (respectively $p < 0.001$, $p = 0.014$, $p = 0.011$). During the COVID-19 pandemic, healthcare workers were exposed to psychological trauma, and their sexual function was negatively affected, with desire mostly unstable or absent.

References

1. Yekefallah L, Mohammadi SD, Namdar P, Moghadam SM, Yekefallah F, Mafi MH. The sexual function, desire, and satisfaction of couples during the outbreak of COVID-19 in Qazvin. Iran J Nurs Midwifery Res. 2023;28(5):544–9.
2. Fuchs A, Matonóg A, Pilarska J, Sieradzka P, Szul M, Czuba B, et al. The impact of COVID-19 on female sexual health. Int J Environ Res. 2020;17:7152.
3. Culha MG, Demir O, Sahin O, Altunrende F. Sexual attitudes of healthcare workers during the COVID-19 epidemic. Int J Impot Res. 2021;33:102–9.
4. Karsiyakali N, Sahin Y, Ates HA, Okucu E, Karabay E. Evaluation of sexual functioning of individuals living in Turkey during the COVID-19 pandemic: a national internet-based survey study. Sex Med. 2021;9:100279.
5. Li G, Tang D, Song B, Wang C, Qunshan S, Xu C, et al. Impact of the COVID-19 pandemic on couple relationships and sexual and reproductive health: a cross-sectional online survey study. J Med Internet Res. 2020;22:e20961.

6. Karagöz MA, Gül A, Borg C, Erihan İB, Uslu M, Ezer M, et al. Influence of the COVID-19 pandemic on sexuality: a cross-sectional study among couples in Turkey. Int J Impot Res. 2020;33:815–23.
7. Cocci A, Giunti D, Tonioni C, Cacciamani G, Tellini R, Polloni G, et al. Love in the time of the COVID-19 pandemic: preliminary results of an online survey conducted during quarantine in Italy. Int J Impot Res. 2020;32:556–7.
8. Brooks SK, et al. The psychological impact of quarantine and how to reduce it: rapid review of the evidence. Lancet. 2020;395:912–20.
9. Presti G, McHugh L, Gloster A, Karekla M, Hayes SC. The dynamics of fear in the time of COVID-19: a contextual perspective of behavioral science. Clin Neuropsychol. 2020;17:65–71.
10. Barlow DH. Causes of sexual dysfunction: the role of anxiety and cognitive interference. J Consult Clin Psychol. 1986;54:140–8.
11. Eleuteri S, Alessi F, Petruccelli F, Saladino V. The global impact of the COVID-19 pandemic on individuals' and couples' sexuality. Front Psychol. 2022 Jan;6(12):798260.
12. Baran O, Aykac A. The effect of fear of COVID-19 transmission on male sexual behavior: a cross-sectional survey study. Int J Clin Pract. 2021;75:e13889. https://doi.org/10.1111/ijcp.13889.
13. Bonato F, Ferreli C, Satta R, Rongioletti F, Atzori L. Syphilis and the COVID-19 pandemic: did the lockdown stop risky sexual behaviors? Clin Dermatol. 2021;39:710–3. https://doi.org/10.1016/j.clindermatol.2020.11.006.
14. Scott-Sheldon LAJ, Mark KP, Balzarini RN, Welling LLM. Call for proposals: special issue of archives of sexual behavior on the impact of COVID-19 on sexual health and behavior. Arch Sex Behav. 2020;49:1393–4. https://doi.org/10.1007/s10508-020-01725-8.
15. Döring N, Walter R. How is the COVID-19 pandemic changing our sexualities? An overview of media narratives in spring 2020. Zeitschrift für Sexualforschung. 2020;33(2):65–75.
16. Gunter J. Coronavirus and sex: questions and answers. New York Times. 2020. Retrieved May 30, 2020 from https://www.nytimes.com/2020/03/30/style/sex-coronavirus-questions-answers.html.
17. Pringels D. How sex workers are coping with the Coronavirus. Vice. 2020. Retrieved May 30, 2020 from https://www.vice.com/en_uk/article/bvg3qq/sex-workers-share-how-coronavirus-is-affecting-their-livelihood.
18. Parmar D, Stavropoulou C, Ioannidis JPA. Health outcomes during the 2008 financial crisis in Europe: a systematic review of the literature. Br Med J. 2016;354:i4588. https://doi.org/10.1136/bmj.i4588.
19. Brooks SK, Webster RK, Smith LE, Woodland L, Wessely S, Greenberg N, Rubin GJ. The psychological impact of quarantine and how to reduce it: rapid review of the evidence. Lancet. 2020;395(10227):912–20. https://doi.org/10.1016/S0140-6736(20)30460-8.
20. Cohan CL, Cole SW. Life course transitions and natural disasters: marriage, birth, and divorce after Hurricane Hugo. J Fam Psychol. 2002;16(1):14–25. https://doi.org/10.1037/0893-3200.16.1.14.
21. Samudyatha UC, Kosambiya JK, Rathore MS. Impact of COVID-19 on profession and health of female sex workers: apprehension, acquiescence, and resilience. Arch Sex Behav. 2024 Jun;53(6):2405–16.
22. Gleason N, Banik S, Braverman J, Coleman E. The impact of the COVID-19 pandemic on sexual behaviors: findings from a National Survey in the United States. J Sex Med. 2021;18(11):1851–62.
23. Gleason N, Banik S, Braverman J, et al. The impact of the COVID-19 pandemic on sexual behaviors: findings from a National Survey in the United States. J Sex Med. 2021;18:1851–62.
24. Global digital population as of April 2022. Available online: https://www.statista.com/statistics/617136/digital-population-worldwide. Accessed 10 May 2022.
25. Getting healthy: the perceived influence of social media on young adult health behaviors. Comput Human Behav. 45, 151–7.
26. Roser M., Ritchie H., Ortiz-Ospina E. Internet. Available online: https://ourworldindata.org/internet. Accessed 10 May 2022.

27. Use of social media during COVID-19 worldwide: statistics and facts. Available online: https://www.statista.com/topics/7863/social-media-use-during-coronavirus-covid-19-worldwide/#dossierKeyfigures. Accessed 10 May 2022.
28. Brown JD, Influences of mass media on sexuality. J Sex Res. 2002;39:42–5. https://doi.org/10.1080/00224490209552118.
29. Luo T, Qin L, Cheng L, Wang S, Zhu Z, Xu J, Chen J, Liu Q, Hu M, Tong J, et al. Determining the cut-off point for the Bergen Social Media Addiction Scale (BSMAS): diagnostic contribution of the six criteria of the addiction component model for social media disorder. J Behav Addict. 2021;10:281–90. https://doi.org/10.1556/2006.2021.00025.
30. Casale S, Akbari M, Seydavi M, Bocci Benucci S, Fioravanti G. Has the prevalence of problematic social media use increased over the past seven years and since the start of the COVID-19 pandemic? A meta-analysis of the studies published since the development of the Bergen social media addiction scale. Addict Behav. 2023;147:107838. https://doi.org/10.1016/j.addbeh.2023.107838. Epub 2023 Aug 23
31. Abedinzadeh M, Vahidi S, Rahavian A, Lojje H, Abouei S. Effect of COVID-19 on the sexual activity of men. Am J Mens Health. 2023;17(4):15579883231193913.
32. Bulut EC, Ertaş K, Bulut D, Koparal MY, Çetin S. The effect of COVID-19 epidemic on the sexual function of healthcare professionals. Andrologia. 2021;53(3):e13971. https://doi.org/10.1111/and.13971. Epub 2021 Jan 13. PMID: 33438223; PMCID: PMC7995045.

Asexuality: Beyond Hypoactive Sexual Desire Disorder?

20

Abstract

Human asexuality is defined as a lack of sexual attraction to anyone or anything. Some studies have suggested that asexuality is an extreme variant of Hypoactive Sexual Desire Disorder (HSDD), a sexual dysfunction characterized by a lack of interest in sex and significant distress.

Keywords

Asexuality · Hypoactive sexual desire disorder · Sexual attraction · Sexual dysfunction · Platonic romantic attraction · Autism · Family genetics

20.1 Introduction

Asexuality has gained increasing attention in academic research and literature over the past year. The study by Carvalho AC et al. [1] for example, focused on the distinction between *romantic asexual individuals, who experience romantic attraction, and aromantic asexual individuals, who do not experience romantic attraction.* A cross-sectional study with members of various online asexual communities (N = 447, 55.02% women; age M = 24.77 years, SD = 7.21) proposed the self-completion of the **Asexuality Identification Scale** to verify sexual behavior and relationships, concerns about sexual performance in a relationship, attachment style.

The results showed that asexual individuals reported a more avoidant attachment style and were more concerned about commitment in the relationship. Conversely, "romantic" asexual individuals reported a lesser aversion to sex, more sexual experiences (both past and current), and more sexual partners in the past.

The study by Lori A. et al. [2] investigated desire, sexual behavior, discomfort related to sex, personality, and psychopathology. The aim was to compare individuals with a score above the limit for asexuality identification (AIS >40) (*n* = 192) with sexual individuals (*n* = 231). The sexual group was further divided into a

E. V. Longhi, *Hypoactive Sexual Desire Disorder*,
https://doi.org/10.1007/978-3-032-00659-2_20

control group ($n = 122$), an HSDD group ($n = 50$) and a group with symptoms of low desire that were not distressing ($n = 59$).

Men in the AIS >40 group were more likely to have never had sexual intercourse, fantasies or previous kisses and caresses compared to all other groups and were less likely to experience sex-related discomfort compared to those with HSDD. For women, those in the HSDD and AIS >40 groups had significantly lower desire compared to the subclinical HSDD and control groups.

Men in the AIS >40 group had significantly lower desire compared to the other three groups. Symptoms of depression were higher among those with subclinical HSDD and HSDD, while there were no group differences in terms of alexithymia or desirable response. This would suggest that asexuality is a sexual dysfunction related to HSDD.

20.2 Psychometric Questionnaires

It is hypothesized that 1% of the adult population is asexual, and research suggests that asexuality is best conceptualized as a sexual orientation. A major limitation in past research on asexuality has been the complete lack of a validated tool to measure asexuality. Due to limitations in recruiting asexual patients, *most studies have relied on recruitment through web-based asexual communities*. This limits the sample to individuals recruited through established asexuality networks/communities.

The study by Yule MA et al. [3] developed and validated ***a self-report questionnaire to assess asexuality***. The questionnaire intended to provide a valid measure regardless of whether the individual identified as asexual and was developed in several stages, including:

1. Development and administration of open-ended questions (209 participants: 139 asexual, and 70 sexual).
2. Administration and analysis of the resulting 111 items (917 participants: 165 asexual, and 752 sexual).
3. Administration and analysis of 37 retained items (1242 participants: 316 asexual, and 926 sexual); and.
4. Validity analysis of the final items.

The resulting Asexuality Identification Scale (AIS), (a 12-item questionnaire), appears to be a brief, valid, and reliable self-assessment tool for the evaluation of asexuality. It is psychometrically valid, easy to administer and has demonstrated the ability to discriminate between sexual and asexual individuals.

Although the lack of sexual attraction, absence of intimate relationships, and self-identification generally define asexuality, there are no unequivocal and certain data. The study by Van Houdenhove E et al. [4] assessed how many patients could be identified as asexual based on each of these criteria and combinations of these criteria.

Participants were recruited through the Asexuality Visibility and Education Network, social media, and posts on various health and lifestyle-related websites.

Five hundred sixty-six participants aged between 18 and 72 years (M = 27.86, SD = 10.53) completed an online survey (24% men, 68.9% women, 7.1% "other"). Based on self-identification or lack of sexual attraction, respectively 71.3% and 69.2% of participants were classified as asexual, while based on the lack of sexual behavior only 48.5% were classified as asexual. Gender differences were found only for those participants who indicated not experiencing sexual attraction, with more women (72.8%) than men (58.8%) indicating a lack of sexual attraction.

Research in China [5] screened models of asexuality in asexual patients according to the parameters: *sexual activities, sexual/romantic attraction, and sexual desire.*

The sample included 227 (64 men and 163 women) asexual participants and 57 (26 men and 31 women) uncertain asexual participants recruited from social networks. The control group included 217 (115 men and 102 women) heterosexual participants recruited from general social networks. Participants with a score equal to or above 40 on the asexuality identification scale were classified as asexual.

Asexual participants reported experiencing low self-eroticism, rare sexual intercourse, minimal or no sexual and romantic attraction compared to heterosexual participants.

This confirms the definition: "people who experience little or no sexual attraction" should be defined as asexual.

Asexual participants scored significantly lower in dyadic sexual desire and slightly lower in solitary sexual desire compared to heterosexual participants.

Significant differences in sexual activities and solitary sexual desire among romantic orientation categories.

Homoromantic participants showed a higher dyadic sexual desire and were more likely to masturbate, indicating heterogeneity among asexual people. The results indicated that Chinese asexual people showed similar patterns of asexuality to those of Western nations. In particular, asexual people have little or no sexual attraction, non-partner-oriented sexual desire, and are heterogeneous in sexual activities and sexual desire. *This implies similar mechanisms underlying the etiology of asexuality across cultures.*

20.3 New Perspectives

In recent years, research has focused on distinguishing between romantic asexual individuals, who experience romantic attraction, and aromantic asexual individuals, who do not experience romantic attraction.

A cross-sectional study [1] with members of various online asexual communities (*N* = 447, 55.02% women; age M = 24.77 years, SD = 7.21) aimed to examine how both groups differed in their identification with the construct of asexuality. *Through the Asexuality Identification Scale individual perspectives on sexuality, sexual behavior and relationships, concerns about commitment and sexual performance in a relationship, and attachment style were studied.*

The results showed that aromantic asexual individuals identified more with asexuality, reported a more avoidant attachment style, and were more concerned about commitment in the relationship. Conversely, romantic asexual individuals reported less aversion to sex, more sexual experiences (both past and current), and more past sexual partners. These individuals also had more frequent romantic relationships—especially in the past—a more intense desire, and a plan to have a romantic relationship in the future (with or without sexual intimacy), and appeared more concerned about sexual performance.

A recent scientific review [6] discussed the findings of 28 relevant studies published in academic journals between January 2020 and July 2022. During this period, academic literature on asexuality mainly focused on:

1. Development of asexual identity.
2. Sex and romantic relationships for asexual individuals.
3. Intersections between asexuality and other aspects of identity.
4. The need for greater awareness and understanding of asexuality.

We could summarize by saying that Asexuality (about 4% of the population) appears to be a generic term that includes demisexuality (experiencing sexual attraction only in the presence of a strong emotional connection) and graysexuality (experiencing sexual attraction only rarely or only under specific circumstances) [7]. The *Asexual Visibility and Education Network*, a network and resource archive on asexuality, defines asexual individuals as those who "are not sexually attracted to people and do not wish to act on attraction to others in a sexual way." Furthermore:—asexual people are more likely to experience anxiety, depression, and other mood disorders compared to people with other sexual orientations. Asexual patients often encounter obstacles in accessing positive and respectful healthcare due to pathologization and misunderstandings. The pathologization of asexuality in healthcare settings has been reported by many asexual patients and can lead to avoidance behaviors of therapies [8]. Arousal and sexual desire refer to the physiological experience of wanting to engage in sexual activity. Attraction concerns the orientation of desire towards specific people. Disorders of arousal and sexual desire refer to a worrying decrease in a person's usual level of arousal and sexual desire. If the person expresses concerns, the practitioner should ask questions to determine if the person lacks attraction, arousal, or sexual desire and to identify their goals [9]. The study of asexuality allows for a better understanding of a little-recognized sexual minority, but also offers a unique opportunity to examine and better understand human sexuality. However, the research has gone deeper. For example, biological factors were considered to evaluate asexuality and compare asexual and allosexual (non-asexual) groups. These studies are part of a growing body of literature that differentiates asexuality from sexual dysfunction and/or psychological disorders. Researchers have used eye-tracking and penile plethysmographs to measure responses to sexual stimuli in cisgender men. By measuring visual attention with eye tracking, researchers found that heterosexual participants had more and longer fixations on erotic images compared to non-erotic images, while asexual participants had more evenly distributed attention. Similarly, a study on sexual arousal found that asexual cisgender men showed lower genital and subjective arousal in response to erotic films compared to allosexual cisgender men (heterosexual and gay). However, asexual and allosexual groups had similar subjective arousal when engaging in sexual fantasies, suggesting that asexuality is not linked to physiological dysfunctions.

20.4 Are Autism Spectrum Disorders and Asexuality Linked?

There is some evidence suggesting that many self-identified asexuals have a formal diagnosis of autism spectrum disorder, which is characterized by deficits in social interaction and communication, as well as restricted and repetitive interests and behaviors. Moreover, the literature shows that asexuality and lack of sexual attraction or low sexual interest are overrepresented in people with autism spectrum disorder compared to neurotypical samples. However, no studies have been conducted to thoroughly investigate the relationship between autism and asexuality. A systematic review of the literature was conducted to examine whether asexuality and autism spectrum disorder are linked. In conclusion, asexuality and autism share various aspects, such as a possible role of prenatal factors; reference to romantic dimensions of sexual attraction and sexual orientation, and non-partner-oriented sexual desire, but future research should explore and clarify this link. Unclear orientation and/or lack of sexual interest have emerged in several studies conducted on ASD samples. In the sample examined by May et al. [10], 21% of girls and 3% of boys in the ASD sample reported uncertainty in sexual attraction. Fernandes et al. [11], examining a cohort of 184 adolescents and young adults (aged between 15 and 39 years) with both low and high functioning ASD, showed a significant prevalence of no evident sexual interest and uncertain sexual orientation. In another study Hellemans et al. [12], 25% of high-functioning autistic adolescents and young adults showed unclear sexual orientation, as reported by their foster home assistants. Similar results were found in a subsequent study conducted by Hellemans et al. [13], in which six individuals with ASD showed unclear sexual orientation, including four with little or no interest in sex. Another interesting finding concerns a significant prevalence of ASD individuals who did not feel the need for a romantic relationship (Strunz et al.) [14], or expressed an absolute disinterest in romantic relationships, physical, intimate, and emotional relationships with others (Cheak-Zamora et al) [15]. The reasons for disinterest in relationships were centered on resistance to intimacy and the fact that relationships could bring "trouble" (Cheak-Zamora et al) [15]. Some ASD individuals have made statements similar to those of asexuals, particularly aromantic asexuals.

The literature suggests that asexuality and autism share various characteristics. If asexuality and ASD share the same etiological factors, such as high exposure to androgens during pregnancy, it would be interesting to investigate this hitherto unknown correlation. In conclusion, evidence of the correlation between asexuality and ASD would have important implications for understanding the sexual behavior of asexual people as well as sexual and romantic functioning in the autistic population. Moreover, a better understanding of this association will likely lead to a broader understanding of the mechanisms that facilitate social connections and attractions among people.

A study by Flanagan SK et al. [16] included 136 adult participants, mainly from the United States, who described themselves as asexual. The participants completed an online survey that contained questions about their experiences with healthcare *providers and doctors*. The results indicated that the majority of participants did not disclose their identity and felt uncomfortable discussing issues related to sexuality with their healthcare providers. Participants who had positive experiences were more likely than those who had negative experiences to indicate that their providers were familiar with asexuality, fully accepted the participant's identity, and responded to the disclosure in a positive and affirming manner.

Positive experiences included providers who informed themselves about asexuality, while negative experiences included *providers who did not believe in the existence of asexuality and between a quarter and half of the participants reported that the providers attributed their asexuality to a health condition*. The results of this study demonstrate the importance of including information on asexual identities in health education and in continuing diversity training in order to increase the cultural sensitivity of healthcare providers.

20.5 Asexuality: What Else Is There to Say?

Following a review of the literature, asexuality has been defined as "*a heterogeneous entity that likely meets the conditions for a sexual orientation and that researchers should further explore the evidence for such categorization*" [17]. The asexual community includes a spectrum of identities; including grayasexual which describes individuals who rarely or only in specific circumstances experience sexual attraction, and demisexual which describes individuals who experience sexual attraction only after an emotional connection [18].

Among the respondents *to the Ace Community Survey*, a large sample [18] of individuals who identify on the ace spectrum, it emerged that those who identified as **asexual** (n = 9476, age M = 22.3, 61.0% women, 12.5% men), **graysexual** (n = 1698, age M = 24.2, 58.8% women, 16.5% men) or **demisexual** (n = 1442, age M = 24.2, 62.8% women, 12.6% men) varied in indicators related to sexual desire, behavior, and identity. Asexual individuals were the least likely to be in a relationship, to experience romantic attraction, or to identify with orientation labels that indicated the genders of attraction such as hetero, bisexual, heteroromantic, and biromantic. Asexual individuals appeared the most likely to identify as aromantic, graysexual individuals were the most likely to identify as grayromantic, and demisexual individuals identified as demiromantic. Asexual individuals also had the lowest scores on measures of sexual desire, personal disposition towards sex, and frequency of masturbation, with graysexual individuals scoring lower than demisexual individuals on the first two.

20.6 Conclusions

People with minority sexual and gender identities (gay, lesbian, bisexual, and transgender) have often been pathologized by healthcare providers and doctors. The premises of the pathologization of asexuality are particularly evident considering that the *lack of sexual desire or interest has been studied in relation to depression, antidepressant medications, and hypothyroidism.*

Indeed, scientific research continues to seek causes that can explain asexuality. One example is the study by Zdaniuk B [19] that investigated the possible prenatal correlates of asexuality. A large international sample ($N = 1634$ women and men) was recruited to explore the associations between sibling composition and asexual sexual orientation ($n = 366$) and to replicate the sibling effects previously reported in individuals with a same-sex attracted orientation ($n = 276$) and a bisexual sexual orientation ($n = 267$) compared to heterosexual individuals ($n = 725$). It was found that a higher overall number of brothers (female fertility effect) predicted a higher likelihood of asexuality in men, and having fewer older sisters and being an only child predicted a higher likelihood of asexuality in women. Regarding same-sex attracted orientations, having a greater number of older sisters increased the likelihood of being a gay man (sororal birth order effect). Having fewer older sisters was associated with a bisexual sexual orientation in women, and a higher overall number of brothers predicted a higher likelihood of bisexuality in men. These results indicate a potential sibling-related contribution to the development of asexuality in women and men, but future studies will need to systematically include clinical experience and patient-reported information. Without criticism or judgment. The study by Andresen JB et al. [20] used baseline questionnaire data on a sample of 62,675 Danes aged between 15 and 89 years, who participated in the Project SEXUS cohort study 2017–2018, to obtain nationally representative estimates of the prevalence of sexual inactivity and dysfunction and to identify their sociodemographic correlates. Overall, it emerged that 23.0% of men with sexual experience and 28.8% of women with sexual experience had not been sexually active with another person in the last year. Sexual inactivity with another person was associated with both young age and old age, single status, less favorable socioeconomic conditions, being underweight and obesity, indicators of poor health, non-consumption of alcohol, and physical inactivity. Among sexually active respondents, 18.0% of men had experienced some dysfunction in the last year, including erectile dysfunction (7.4%), premature ejaculation dysfunction (10.0%), orgasmic dysfunction (4.0%), and/or genital pain dysfunction (0.7%). Among women, 20.4% experienced some dysfunction in the last year, including lubrication dysfunction (9.1%), orgasmic dysfunction (12.2%), genital pain dysfunction (5.0%), and/or vaginal cramp dysfunction (vaginismus) (0.8%). Furthermore, 3.4% of men and 9.9% of women with a spouse/partner experienced a hypoactive sexual desire disorder in the previous 4 weeks. Using the International Index of Erectile Function (IIEF-5) 5-item and the Female Sexual Function Index 6-item (FSFI-6) among respondents with a spouse or partner who had attempted sexual intercourse in the last 4 weeks, it was found that 3.8% of men experienced moderate or severe erectile dysfunction (IIEF-5 score $\leq$ 11) and 20.8% of women experienced some sexual dysfunction (FSFI-6 score $\leq$ 19) during that period. Single status, difficulties in paying bills, and, among men, unemployment were positively associated with sexual dysfunction. In conclusion, various sociodemographic disparities in the prevalence of sexual inactivity and dysfunction in Denmark were more common among singles and those reporting financial difficulties.

References

1. Carvalho AC, Rodrigues DL. Sexuality, sexual behavior, and relationships of asexual individuals: differences between aromantic and romantic orientation. Arch Sex Behav. 2022;51(4):2159–68.
2. Brotto LA, Yule MA, Gorzalka BB. Asexuality: an extreme variant of sexual desire disorder? J Sex Med. 2015;12(3):646–60.
3. Yule MA, Brotto LA, Gorzalka BB. A validated measure of no sexual attraction: the asexuality identification scale. Psychol Assess. 2015;27(1):148–60.
4. Van Houdenhove E, Gijs L, T'Sjoen G, Enzlin P. Asexuality: a multidimensional approach. J Sex Res. 2015;52(6):669–78.
5. Zheng L, Su Y. Patterns of asexuality in China: sexual activity, sexual and romantic attraction, and sexual desire. Arch Sex Behav. 2018;47(4):1265–76.
6. Hille JJ. Beyond sex: a review of recent literature on asexuality. Curr Opin Psychol. 2023;49:101516. ISSN 2352-250X.
7. Schneckenburger SA, Tam MWY, Ross LE. Asexual competent practices in healthcare: a narrative review. J Gay Lesbian Ment Health. 2023:314.
8. Foster AB, Scherrer KS. Clients identified as asexual in clinical settings: implications for culturally competent practice. Psychol Sex Orientat Gend Divers. 2014;1:422–30.
9. Bogaert AF. Asexuality: what it is and why it's important. J Sex Res. 2015;52:362–79.
10. May T, Pang KC, Williams K. Brief report: sexual attraction and relationships in adolescents with autism. J Autism Dev Disord. 2017;47(6):1910–6.
11. Fernandes LC, Gillberg CI, Cederlund M, Hagberg B, Gillberg C, Billstedt E. Aspects of sexuality in adolescents and adults diagnosed with autism spectrum disorders in childhood. J Autism Dev Disord. 2016;46(9):3155–65.
12. Hellemans H, Colson K, Verbraeken C, Vermeiren R, Deboutte D. Sexual behavior in high-functioning male adolescents and young adults with autism spectrum disorder. J Autism Dev Disord. 2007;37(2):260–9.
13. Hellemans H, Roeyers H, Leplae W, Dewaele T, Deboutte D. Sexual behavior in male adolescents and young adults with autism spectrum disorder and borderline/mild mental retardation. Sex Disabil. 2010;28(2):93–104.
14. Strunz S, Schermuck C, Ballerstein S, Ahlers CJ, Dziobek I, Roepke S. Romantic relationships and relationship satisfaction among adults with Asperger syndrome and high-functioning autism. J Clin Psychol. 2017;73(1):113–25.
15. Cheak-Zamora NC, Teti M, Maurer-Batjer A, O'Connor KV, Randolph JK. Interests, knowledge, and sexual and relational experiences among adolescents and young adults with autism spectrum disorder. Arch Sex Behav. 2019;48(8):2605–15.
16. Flanagan SK, Peters HJ. Asexual-identified adults: interactions with health-care practitioners. Arch Sex Behav. 2020 Jul;49(5):1631–43.
17. Brotto LA, Yule M. Asexuality: sexual orientation, paraphilia, sexual dysfunction, or none of the above? Arch Sex Behav. 2017;46:619–27. https://doi.org/10.1007/s10508-016-0802-7.

18. Copulsky D, Hammack PL. Asexuality, graysexuality, and demisexuality: distinctions in desire, behavior, and identity. J Sex Res. 2023;60:221–30. https://doi.org/10.1080/00224499.2021.2012113.
19. Zdaniuk B, Milani S, Makarenko B, Marriott N, Bogaert AF, Brotto LA. Asexuality: its relationship to sibling sex composition and birth order. Arch Sex Behav. 2024;54:51.
20. Andresen JB, Graugaard C, Andersson M, Bahnsen MK, Frisch M. Sexual inactivity and dysfunction in Denmark: a project SEXUS study. Arch Sex Behav. 2022;51(8):3669–88. https://doi.org/10.1007/s10508-022-02348-x. Epub 2022 Sep 20.